The 10-Minute Total Body Breakthrough

BY SEAN FOY, M.A.

WITH NELLIE SABIN AND MIKE SMOLINSKI

FOREWORD BY WILLIAM SEARS, M.D.

WORKMAN PUBLISHING · NEW YORK

Library of Congress Cataloging-in-Publication Data is available.
ISBN 978-0-7611-5419-8

Cover and interior photographs copyright © 2009 by James Maciariello

Additional photos credits:
Erika Nungaray p. 8, 9, 10, 11, 12, 13; SPRI Products, Inc. (www.spri.com) p. 135, 136, 137 (top), 148 (top), 160 (top), 171 (top), 184, 185, 186, 187 (top), 199 (top), 212 (top), 222; Andrew Terzes (www.terzesphoto.com) p. 271, 273, 274, 276, 277, 281, 283, 285

Art Direction: Janet Vicario
Design: Lidija Tomas

Workman books are available at special discounts when purchased in bulk for premiums and sales promotions as well as for fund-raising or educational use. Special editions of book excerpts can also be created to specification. For details, contact the Special Sales Director at the address below.

Workman Publishing Company, Inc.
225 Varick Street
New York, NY 10014-4381
www.workman.com

Printed in China

First printing September 2009
10 9 8 7 6 5 4 3 2 1

To the love of my life:
Joanne,
the greatest person I know

NOTE: Please consult a physician before beginning this exercise program—particularly if you have ever had a heart attack or been diagnosed with cardiovascular or coronary heart disease, have frequent chest pains or often feel faint or dizzy upon physical exertion, have high blood pressure or high cholesterol levels, diabetes, liver or kidney disease, are female less than 6 months postpartum, or are under 18 years of age. In addition, ask for your doctor's advice if you have muscle, joint or bone problems that might be aggravated by exercise.

CONTENTS

The Breakthrough

I first met Sean Foy in 1998 when I needed a personal trainer to help me get out of my metabolic mess after surgery, radiation and chemotherapy for colon cancer. Many of my friends had tried workout programs that were so time-consuming they couldn't stick with them, but Sean showed me a different way. A master motivator, he introduced me to a new kind of math: Invest 10 minutes a day in your body and, in return, end up feeling better and living longer. This was something I could do—and something I *have* done for more than 10 years now.

Sean became not only my personal trainer, but my friend, fitness mentor and coauthor of *Dr. Sears' LEAN Kids Book.* I'm a "show me the science" type of doctor—our bodies are far too valuable to be submitted to fad diets and unscientifically tested programs—and Sean was always ready with the answers. You'll see what I mean as you read this book, since he's woven frequent science boxes into his text to prove the soundness of the 10-Minute Total Body Breakthrough. But just in case there are any doubters left, he follows them up with many of his personal success stories, of which I am one.

I'm happy to report that Sean's program chanced my life. At age 65, I applied to upgrade my life insurance policy, which required a thorough physical exam. A week later, I got a call from one of the insurance company's doctors, who initially shocked me by saying "The computer rejected your application because your cholesterol was too high." Before I had time to complain, he explained: "The reason is, your *good* cholesterol is unusually high. Besides, we seldom see such a healthy cholesterol profile in a person of your age. What are you doing to stay so fit?" I told him—after he assured me that my insurance application was approved—that the answer was LEAN: Change your *L*ifestyle, *E*xercise, *A*ttitude and *N*utrition. I also informed him that, even though I had the blood chemistry profile of a much younger person, I was taking no regular prescription medicines. Thank you, Sean Foy!

When patients ask me for a quick and easy fitness program that they can make a lasting part of their lives, I write them this prescription from The 10-Minute Total Body Breakthrough:

- 4 minutes of high-energy aerobic training

- 3 minutes of resistance exercise

- 2 minutes of core-strengthening exercises

- 1 minute of stretching and deep breathing

"Wow, I can do that!" my patients say. But the right workout for *you* is the one you will do. The 10-Minute Total Body Breakthrough is a routine *anyone* can do—no matter how pressed for time. It makes so much sense to me. Just as we focus on eating nutrient-dense foods, those that pack the most nutrition into the fewest calories, we should be focusing on getting the most fitness benefit from our workouts. In other words, we should be getting more bang for our exercise buck. By packing his years of fitness-training experience into a total body breakthrough that can be accomplished in just 10 minutes, Sean has made that possible.

Another thing I especially like about this book is that it focuses on not only a makeover of the body but of the mind. You will enjoy the voice of Sean the marriage and family counselor as he explains that relationship fitness is like physical fitness—if you don't work to build it, it atrophies.

This is a book for all ages. One of the first things to "go" when we get older is our muscle mass. It's the "use it or lose it" principle. Muscle loss starts a downward spiral: move less and lose muscle, the body's number one calorie burner; gain body fat, get frail, fall more; get cardiovascular disease, diabetes and Alzheimer's from too much excess body fat; need more medicines to help the three big Ds—diabetes, dementia and cardiovascular disease—and many more disabilities. Because you don't feel well, you don't move well, and the spiral continues on down. The 10-Minute Total Body Breakthrough program keeps this from happening. "I don't have time for exercise," you may counter. Then you better reserve more time for the hospital. "But I don't *like* exercising!" Do you like hurting?

Many of the exercises in this program, especially at Level I, can be done anytime, anywhere, using your body as the weight and resistance to safely work up to a program of free weights. The flip cards at the back of the book allow you to mix and match exercises to fit your personal fitness level and daily schedule, guaranteeing that you progress instead of regress. And the program doesn't stop there. We're introduced to a healthy and lasting dietary plan that boils down to three words: *Eat real foods.* I'm happy that Sean takes the fads out of dieting to really keep off the fat. Instead of *low-fat* diets, think *right fats;* instead of *low carbs,* think *right carbs.* What we learn in this book is that it's not the *quantity* of food that counts; it's the *quality.* Here's where Sean makes a very important point: Being thin is not the same as being fit.

In developing the LEAN Start Program together, Sean and I shared a common motivation: we enjoy what in medicine we call a helper's high. By helping others go from fat to fit and from sad to happy for a measly investment of 10 minutes a day, we feel better ourselves—and this is a priceless feeling.

I wish you good reading and good health!

William Sears, M.D.

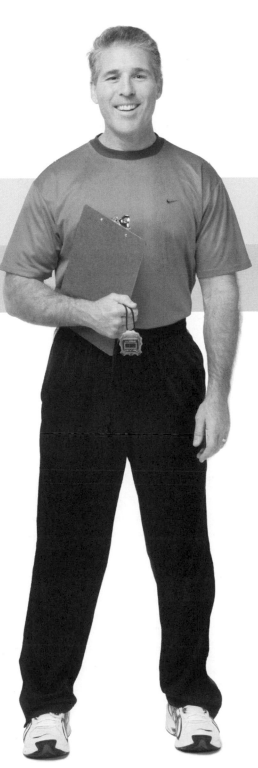

Do You Have 10 Minutes?

4
3
2
1

It's About Time!

Countdown to a New You

Yes, it *is* about time. It's *all* about time. How does it fly by so fast? Where does it go? Working, shopping, putting meals on the table, raising kids, doing housework, getting to appointments, volunteering, taking care of aging parents—all these responsibilities keep us on the run. And if we find some free time, we don't want to spend it on a treadmill.

The fact is, we're just too busy to squeeze the same old time-consuming fitness regimens into our schedules. What's needed is a new approach to exercise, a way to achieve maximum results in the shortest amount of time possible: fitness at the speed of life. And that's exactly what *The 10-Minute Total Body Breakthrough* is all about. When you follow the guidelines in this book, packing every type of exercise into just 10 minutes, you *will* develop the fit body you never had time for before. And once you become more fit, your life will change in more ways than you can imagine.

It's true! You can be in the best shape of your life by exercising just 10 minutes a day. And as you'll see in the pages of this book, I have the research, published studies, statistics and personal case histories to prove it.

It All Started with a Football Injury . . .

Back when I was a sophomore in college, I blew out my knee playing football and had to live with my left leg in a cast for eight long weeks. At first, the cast felt really tight and uncomfortable. One of the worst parts was having an itch that I'd have to scratch by sliding a coat hanger down between the cast and my skin. But then the muscles began to atrophy, and after a while I could reach down inside with my hand to scratch my leg. By the time the cast came off, I had one strong leg and one skinny leg that looked like it belonged to an old man. I couldn't bend that leg or stand on it. In fact, I could barely move it. Chronologically, my left leg was 19; physically, it was 90.

But what started out feeling like total misfortune turned out to be a blessing. I became very interested in the way the body recovers from a sports injury. I threw myself into rebuilding my leg muscles. And I learned all I could about healing.

After graduating with a B.S. in exercise physiology, I applied for a position as a "behavioral health specialist." I wasn't exactly sure what that meant, but I knew a lot about health and a little about behavior—and I got the job. As it turned out, I was responsible for getting people to lose weight by following a strict diet using meals premade by a certain well-known company. I loved working one-on-one with my dieters and helping them achieve their target weights. Victory! Success! And then . . . trouble. My dieters could not successfully make the transition to eating real food. Inevitably, the pounds came back, and I couldn't help wondering if the company truly wanted people to lose weight for good—or did it want people to keep re-gaining so they would keep spending money on its weight-loss meals?

I decided to focus full-time on helping people get healthy, and after working as a personal trainer for five years I started my own company, Personally Fit. As I had seen in my first job, most people had neglected their health and fitness for years, and now they wanted to lose six pounds in a week or drop four sizes in a month. These people had what's called a Band-Aid mentality—they would fix their weight problems quickly with crash dieting and a little exercise, then resume living as before. They were forgetting that *thin* is not the same as *fit*.

A Change of Tune: Annie to the Rescue

I started addressing larger groups about health and fitness, advising people to incorporate regular exercise into their lives, to eat their fruits and vegetables, to try harder, to plan better, to fit it all in. But I began to see a glassy look on the faces in the audience. And then, one evening, I noticed a woman who clearly was not going along with me. I'll call her Annie. I tried to ignore her, but she was like a little black cloud, sitting with her head down in the front row. I went on talking about the benefits of exercise. I showed slides about the fat content of fast food. I told funny stories. I was encouraging and upbeat, but Annie would have none of it.

After my presentation, Annie came up to me and said, "I want you to know I've tried everything— every pill, every potion, every diet and every exercise program. I know what I'm supposed to do, and I can do it for a little while, but I have lost the same 60 pounds over and over again. I just don't know where to turn anymore."

I searched my brain for the right response, but nothing came. I knew the standard "do more, do better" speech wasn't going to work, and for once I was at a loss for words. After all, what can you say to someone who has tried everything?

Who Has Time for Exercise?

As time went on, I could not get Annie out of my head. She had come to me for help, and I had failed her. I wondered how many other Annies were sitting in the audience. Was that glassy look a way of saying, "*Are you nuts? We barely have time to get to the bathroom, let alone put aside an hour for exercise. We already know we need to exercise more and eat better. Tell us how to do it while we're juggling our busy schedules and responsibilities!*"

I began to realize that the number one barrier to experiencing long-lasting transformation was the age-old dilemma: How do you invest in yourself and still keep everything else going? For most people, working out was long, boring and arduous, and they had plenty of other things to do. When I talked about weight training and cardiovascular exercise, what they were hearing was "blah, blah, blah." They were far too busy to exercise or prepare healthy meals. Going to a gym would use up an hour or an hour and a half of precious time they could be spending with their family. Exercising meant less time to pick up the dry cleaning, buy birthday presents, get groceries, take the dog to the vet, get a haircut, visit a grandparent in the nursing home or see a cousin in the hospital. An hour on the treadmill meant less time for paying bills, checking e-mail, making phone calls and preparing presentations. It even meant less time to relax—to just kick back, watch the game, read a book, go out to dinner or catch a movie. For people who set their alarm clocks earlier in the morning in order to work out, exercising even took time away from sleeping!

By now, I had a family of my own. I had married my high school sweetheart, Joanne, and we had a two-year-old son named Joel; our daughter, Brooke, was soon to come. I was juggling a new business and a new home life, and I knew firsthand all about time and lack of sleep. I decided I needed help finding the right answers. My thinking was: I spend all day helping people improve their physical health and fitness, working on their bodies, but I need to address the mental and emotional aspects of their health; lasting change involves much more than just exercising and healthy eating. I attended graduate school and eventually received a master's degree in marriage and family counseling. My master's thesis was on the subject of whole-person health—physical, emotional, relational and spiritual.

Small Efforts Add Up

I remember one behavioral counseling class in which the professor, Dr. Joe, asked: "What is the one thing an individual can do to destroy a relationship, without fail?" We were all puzzled by the question, but different students ventured their answers. Argue too much? Be disrespectful? But the right answer was "Nothing." When nothing intentional is done to build a relationship, it atrophies and dies. Conversely, small, consistent efforts can restore a relationship back to health. Over time, these acts build more trust, then greater confidence and, finally, enthusiasm. Even the smallest of efforts, over time, can yield significant results.

Now I asked myself, *What is the one thing people can do to destroy their health?* The answer: *Nothing.* Without physical activity, muscles literally shrink, like my leg when it was in a cast. And weight begins to creep up. Stairs are too much effort, so we take the elevator. We do less and less, and get bigger and softer. By the time our fitness problem becomes obvious, fixing it seems overwhelming—unless we begin to take the first small steps toward success.

Fast Fitness:
A New Kind of Workout

started to work with organizations other than health clubs, knowing that every company would benefit from offering my exercise program to its employees. It was a win-win situation. The employees would become healthier and happier, and the company would have a more productive workforce—with fewer expensive medical claims and employee sick days.

My first corporate client, Nutrilite, signed up employees for 15-minute Health Breaks. I would need a speedy workout for them, and I wondered what would happen if I took a complete exercise program and broke it down into smaller steps. What if I asked them to do *less* instead of more? I started asking people what they thought of exercising for shorter periods. I would say, "Hey, if you could see the same results in a third of the time, would you be interested?" People usually answered, "Are you kidding me? Bring it on!"

I examined dozens of fitness plans to see if anyone else had a worthy approach to fast fitness. I knew my criteria. My plan had to include cardiovascular exercise, strength training, core-strengthening exercises (for the muscles of the abdomen, lower back and hips), stretching and deep breathing—all in a short amount of time. It also needed a sound, simple nutrition component that would put an end to yo-yo dieting, a plan people could follow for a lifetime of healthy eating. I found nothing. It looked like it was up to me to create "the perfect program."

4·3·2·1 and the "No Diet" Diet

At just about this time, I had the privilege of meeting Dr. William Sears, the renowned American pediatrician who has written dozens of parenting books with his wife, Martha. As we collaborated on the book *LEAN Kids,* a program designed to combat the juvenile obesity epidemic, I researched the kinds of activities that kids like and dislike. They enjoy stop-and-start games like dodgeball and tag, which combine periods of intense exercise with periods of moderate activity or rest. They like whole-body activities such as running, swimming and using the monkey bars on the playground. They naturally combine activities to utilize their entire bodies. For example, hopscotch combines hopping (which strengthens the legs) and throwing (which engages the upper body). Like most adults, children do not like to work out—to go for long jogs or walk on a treadmill. However, if you're a kid, bicycling up a steep hill to a friend's house is fun and just happens to be a fine cardiovascular workout.

Now I began to wonder, what if I encouraged my new clients to exercise more like kids? Could I make exercise fun again? Could I structure a workout around periods of intense activity alternating with slower periods for catching your breath?

I discovered that articles were appearing in professional journals about a new approach to exercise: interval or "burst" training. Studies showed that intermittent high-intensity exercise was as beneficial as long workouts. Exercise did not have to be prolonged, painful or boring to strengthen muscles, burn calories and provide a post-workout metabolic boost. This was good news for people who were intimidated by the time and energy required for most exercise regimens. I started to assemble a new kind of workout from the ground up.

■ What if I asked people to perform **4 minutes** of higher-intensity cardiovascular activity? Anybody can do 4 minutes!

- What if I asked them to do **3 minutes** of strengthening exercises for their entire body?

- What if I could get them to tone and strengthen the muscles of their abdomen, lower back and hips for just **2 minutes**?

- And what if I then added **1 minute** of stress-reducing stretching and deep breathing?

The result would be a revolutionary 10-minute total body workout, something the fitness industry had never seen before—a program that would let *everyone* meet his or her fitness goals.

I knew that along with this new exercise regimen, people would need to learn a new way to eat. With so much contradictory nutrition and diet information out there, my new clients would be confused about what approach is best. *LEAN Kids* included a system called "traffic light" eating, based on the Stoplight Diet created in the 1970s by Dr. Leonard Epstein at the University of Buffalo. Using this approach to healthy eating, foods are divided into three groups: "green light" (go ahead!), "yellow light" (use caution) and "red light" (stop and think before you eat). This is a simple system that any age group can follow. For my clients, it would mean no more diets or calorie counting, no more cycles of deprivation and guilt, no more fat clothes and skinny clothes. Just a solid eating plan for life.

The 10-Minute Total Body Breakthrough program is based on a combination of 4•3•2•1 workouts and healthy eating. You're about to discover, as my corporate clients did, that it's simple, it's fast . . . and it works.

Success Begets Success

I love going to work every day because I *know* I am helping others. I feel it's a privilege for me to be able to speak with people, heart to heart, about what they really want to accomplish and to encourage them step by step as they take their personal journey into fitness. Again and again, I see people transform their bodies and their lives, and I never get tired of it.

For example, Michelle started the 4•3•2•1 workouts because she wanted to be an energetic mom who could keep up with her three kids. Now she's less tired, needs less sleep and is able to have more fun with her children. She can haul around her five-year-old effortlessly, and at a roller skating party she was one of the few moms who actually got out and skated. But Michelle has discovered yet another reason to make healthy lifestyle changes. Her children have started to model her behavior, which motivates her to do her best. Michelle says, "My kids are really excited about what I'm doing. They want to get involved. When I do my workout, they'll say, 'Wait, Mommy, let me do it with you!' So it's a great way for them to start establishing healthy habits, too. I am so glad I made this commitment to myself and to my kids. It has truly changed my life."

Many people assume that being out of shape is just part of getting old. Not so! Before Carol started using the 4•3•2•1 workouts, she felt her life was out of whack, and she wondered if she was too old to turn things around. "There are four things in life you have to have in balance—faith, family, finances and fitness," she says. "And the fitness part was totally out of whack for me!" Now Carol has her balance back, plus a lot more energy. "You know what?" she adds. "You can begin anything anytime—even after 40!"

When Jacki first started to use the 4•3•2•1 workouts, her focus was to lose weight and look better. After nine weeks, she said: "I'm down two sizes, and I'm looking in the mirror and thinking, *Whoa, that's much better!*" However, becoming more fit brought other changes Jacki never expected. "Now I just love the way I feel. Plus, I've added a lot more self-discipline into other areas of my life," she explains. "Not just eating and exercise, but getting things done. I'm becoming more of a scheduled person. And I'm prioritizing. I'm seeing what's important in my life. I'm more focused on my life and on what counts. I don't let the things that seem to be so urgent take over. I'm not going back. I expect in 10 years to be a different person."

Greg is one of the participants who appreciate how increased fitness can lead to business success. "It has changed my whole life," he says. "For a while there, everything was stiff and I couldn't move. Now I'm playing tennis with my family and shooting baskets—and that's just the beginning. I'll tell you something, feeling better turns into dollars. When you feel better, you can make more money!"

4·3·2·1 Success Stories

Thousands of people, from Maine to Australia, have experienced the benefits of the 4•3•2•1 program over the last six years. Meeting and working with them has been my privilege, and now I'd like you to get to know some of them in more depth. These individuals—like you—have families, jobs, businesses to run, all the stresses of life, and yet they managed to recapture their health and fitness . . . all at the speed of life.

Dinah's Story:
Family Fitness

As a business strategist, Dinah travels at least every other week. She had always been athletic and trim, but after reaching a certain age she realized she was slowly putting on a pound or two a year. It added up to some extra weight she simply was not happy about. Just at the point when she started to buy loose-fitting clothes, Dinah signed up for the 4•3•2•1 program.

Dinah appreciated the fact that she did not have to go to a gym to do the 10-minute workouts. This made it easier for her to keep up with her exercise when she was on the road. She had always eaten healthy foods, but she added more fresh vegetables and fish to her diet, ate fewer carbs and watched her portion sizes more carefully. She also started eating breakfast, and this change alone gave her more energy and made it possible for her to go through an entire day without calorie-rich snacking. Dinah lost over 20 pounds. And months after she started the program, she ran a half-marathon—without even feeling sore the next day!

Dinah has been on the 4•3•2•1 program for several years, and she remains highly motivated professionally as well as personally. Her husband works out regularly, her three sons and their wives are all fitness buffs, and even her active grandchildren eat healthy snacks. Dinah is an extremely energetic grandma, and her extended family is the picture of fitness.

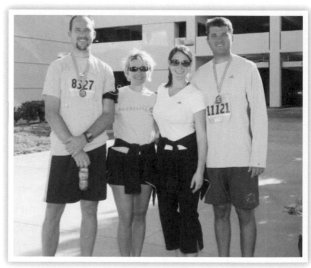

Dinah (second from left) lost 20 pounds and ran a half-marathon to celebrate.

Frank's Story:
Defeating Diabetes

When you see New Frank, you could never imagine what Old Frank was like. These days, Frank is energetic and athletic. He runs long-distance races, has gotten into bicycling and is thinking about starting to bike the 12 miles to and from work. You'd never guess that Old Frank got exhausted every day and had significant back problems.

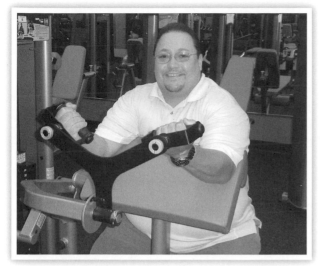

Frank got his diabetes under control with diet and exercise.

Frank is a packaging engineer—a position that requires him to wake up at 4:30 each morning and keeps him away from home until 5:00 or 6:00 in the evening. In the old days, Frank would eat dinner very late and then go to bed. He was tired in the mornings and couldn't imagine finding time for exercise. He drank soda all day and had no idea that his poor food choices were abusing his body. He tried some crash diets, but without success.

Frank received a life-altering shock when his doctor told him he had diabetes; his blood sugar was 300 (well above normal). The doctor immediately started Frank on two medications and told him what would happen to his health if he didn't get his weight and blood sugar under control. It wasn't good! As it happened, the 4•3•2•1 program was being offered where Frank worked. Knowing that exercise could help him control his diabetes, Frank was extremely motivated; in 10 weeks he lost 17 pounds and 10% body fat!

Frank appreciated the 4•3•2•1 program because it was a small time commitment that yielded big results. Little by little, he transitioned into his new lifestyle. He gave up soda and alcohol and started drinking plenty of water. He ate less "white food"— things like pasta, potatoes and white bread—and increased his fruits and vegetables. He cut out the late-night eating, and now, when he gets hungry, he just eats more salad. Today Frank no longer suffers from back pain. He takes walks every evening. And most important, his diabetes is under control. This is an accomplishment that few people manage. "It's a huge weight off my back," he says. "My doctor was so impressed when my blood sugar dropped down to 100—and even more so that I've maintained it just with diet and exercise. I've been medication-free ever since."

Zenaida's Story:
Who's Laughing Now?

Zenaida is a senior pharmaceutical technician, and her job involves working with heavy bags, boxes and drums of ingredients, plus weighing the powders that go into the company's products. Zenaida works 12-hour shifts and has been on the job for 19 years. She has two teenagers, and her husband, a truck driver, is often away.

Before she started the 4•3•2•1 program, Zenaida was often tired during the day and in the evening. She had no time for exercise, and her eating habits— traditional home-cooked Hispanic meals with plenty of starches and high-fat fried food—were not doing her any favors. Her doctor wanted her to take medicine to combat her elevated cholesterol levels. Zenaida realized she wasn't getting any younger or

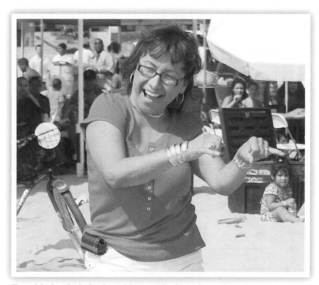

Zenaida is glad she lost 28 pounds, but she enjoys her husband's compliments best of all.

any healthier. *If something happens to me,* she wondered, *what happens to my kids?*

When Zenaida joined the 4•3•2•1 Challenge at work, she began exercising at home. At first, she couldn't finish a single workout. Her teenagers would walk by and giggle. But she persisted, and her kids soon became interested in what she was doing.

Zenaida realized for the first time that what you eat can actually hurt you. She turned her cooking and eating habits upside down. Little by little, she cut out junk food, and she started to cook more chicken. She added salmon to the family menu, chose salad over tortillas and started watching her portion sizes.

Zenaida also learned for the first time that the numbers on her bathroom scale did not indicate how fit she was. She became discouraged about not losing more weight, and was ready to quit when she learned that her new muscle mass was offsetting her loss of fat. Today Zenaida says, "The scale, for me, doesn't mean anything. I know I'm more fit because of the way my clothes fit. It looks like I bought all new uniforms!"

In five months, Zenaida lost 28 pounds and lowered her blood pressure, cholesterol levels and percentage of body fat. Today she goes to the gym, where she does kickboxing, yoga, running, swimming and stair-stepping, and takes "boot camp" exercise classes for fun. What's more, her kids are now going to the gym with her! Zenaida even goes running with her nieces and nephews, and beats kids half her age.

Says Zenaida: "Our lives are very stressful. We really have to take care of ourselves, and the 4•3•2•1 program got me on track." Today she feels stronger and more confident, and her naturally cheerful personality is back. She adds so much energy and good cheer to the workplace that people miss her when she's not there. Best of all are her husband's compliments: "They're better than any trophy!"

Bert's Story:
A Lucky Nosebleed

After trying to ignore a nosebleed that lasted for days, Bert finally went to the emergency room. To his surprise, the doctors flew into action. Bert was quickly

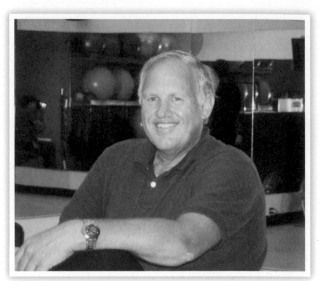

Bert lost 85 pounds . . . and he's getting married!

hooked up to wires, machines and monitors. It turned out his blood pressure was out of control at 230/185 and he could have had a stroke at any moment.

Other than having a red face, Bert had no indications that he was in trouble. High blood pressure is called a "silent killer" because of its lack of symptoms. A formerly active guy who loved to surf and ski, he knew he had gotten heavier. Bert now had a stressful desk job as a supervisor for the custodial department of two facilities, and he did not have the energy to take on any additional responsibilities. Since he lived alone, he found it easier to stop for fast food than to cook for himself. And every day he drank two containers of his favorite beverage: the 44-ounce Super Big Gulp soda from 7-Eleven.

The day after Bert was released from the hospital, he signed up for the 4•3•2•1 program at work. "If you'd told me that in two years I'd be running marathons, I'd have told you that you were nuts," Bert says today. Now he's a fitness role model. As of this writing, he has dropped over 85 pounds and his blood pressure is down to 135/80. With his increased energy level and his blood pressure under control, Bert has a new, positive attitude. Everyone at work comments on how different he is. He has taken on new duties at work and has become more outgoing and fun-loving. He is no longer living in isolation, and he enjoys the camaraderie at sporting events. He's even getting married. And his next goal is to run the New York City marathon—which I am certain he will. Once you find your inner athlete, anything can happen!

Jean's Story:
More Time to Be Mom

As a process engineer, Jean works up to 12 hours a day. She is also a single mother of two teenagers who not only need help buying school clothes, help with homework and help with last-minute school projects, but also participate in dance class, drawing class, marching band, music lessons, cross-country, Chinese school and—oh, yes—helping the homeless.

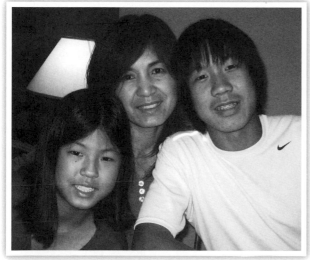

Jean (center) now has more time to spend with her two active teenage kids.

Jean had tried to lose weight for years, but at just 122 pounds it wasn't easy. Exercise did not appeal to her, and she had no energy and no time for working out. With 4•3•2•1, Jean finally found a fast way to exercise and to change her body composition. She forced herself to attend the company 4•3•2•1 workout sessions and cut back on her beloved homemade desserts. As Jean puts it, "You have to give up something to gain something."

Jean lost seven pounds of fat, gained muscle and along the way also acquired a brand-new energy level that stunned her coworkers and her kids. Today, as

a 4•3•2•1 ambassador, she's always trying to get her colleagues to go to workouts with her. "Come on," she says. "It'll be good for you!"

Now when Jean gets home, she has the energy to hang out with her kids. She can run errands for them, and they keep asking, "You're not too tired?" They're getting better grades, and Jean's relationship with them has changed dramatically. Before, Jean was too tired to hear about their day—she had to go straight to bed to make it through the next day. Recently they told her, "We didn't know you cared." Now they know.

Angel's Story:
From Skeptic to Believer

Angel, an avid exerciser for years, was very skeptical about the 4•3•2•1 program. But since he wasn't satisfied with the results of his workouts, he thought he'd give 4•3•2•1 training a go. Now he's glad he put his skepticism aside: "The 4•3•2•1 workouts have done what many previous training programs have not been able to do."

Specifically, Angel no longer requires the medication he took for two years to lower his blood pressure, since his numbers dropped to well below average. His resting heart rate also dropped from 90 to 56 beats per minute. And his thyroid and liver blood work results, which had been abnormal prior to the program, are now just fine.

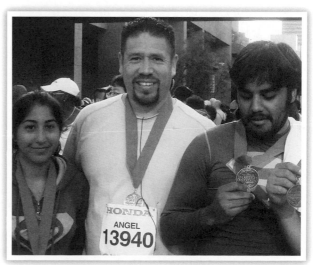

Angel took 35 minutes off his marathon time.

Although Angel had been working out for some time, he still struggled with his energy levels and stamina. Today, after doing the 4•3•2•1 program, he reports that he can sustain physical activity for much longer periods without feeling out of breath. He recently ran the Los Angeles marathon, beating last year's time by a full 35 minutes. He couldn't walk for weeks after his first marathon, but this year he was sore for only one day. He gives the credit to 4•3•2•1 training!

Tom's Story:
From One Step at a Time to One State at a Time

Before 4•3•2•1, Tom had never seen the inside of a gym. He was neither fat nor fit. He carried a few extra pounds but did not appear heavy. Tom had played tennis when he was younger, but between the time he spent with his family and time at his job, he no longer had any opportunity for exercise.

When 4•3•2•1 was offered at the company where he worked, Tom made up his mind to improve his fitness. He started walking, then jogging, then running. Before long, he was running marathons. Tom lost weight, changed his percentage of body fat and lowered his cholesterol by 20 points. He has so much more energy that he changed from a sedentary job to one that requires walking.

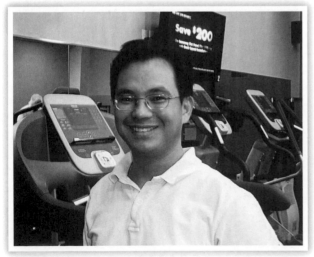

Tom was never fat, but now he's *fit*.

In the old days, Tom generally skipped breakfast and would eat at McDonald's a couple of times a week. Today, when he eats a red-light food, he thinks, *How many laps will I have to do to make up for this?*

Tom's new fitness level has had a huge effect on his relationships. He has become an inspiration to his colleagues. He says that running gets rid of his stress, so he has a more positive outlook and can enjoy his family after work. Today, his personal goal is to run a marathon in all 50 states. He says, "It will be a cheap way to see the country!"

My Personal 4·3·2·1 Superstars

I can't resist sharing two more stories with you. The following individuals are important to me personally and professionally, and they have taken 4•3•2•1 to a level that is achieved by few. Without discussing their chronological ages, let's just say these two can run circles around men and women twice as young. They are an inspiration to me.

Diane's Story:
From Strong to Stronger

I have worked closely with Diane for over 15 years. Diane has a husband, Rich, and three daughters who are college athletes. A talented fitness coach, Diane holds many positions in the industry. She is a corporate wellness manager, a master fitness instructor and a private trainer; she teaches many different types of fitness class in health clubs; and she was one of the first people to teach 4•3•2•1 classes in our corporate programs. Today, Diane certifies 4•3•2•1 instructors, coaches the participants in the "A New Way to a New You" program (see Chapter 11) and travels extensively to give seminars.

Diane formerly had an office job, and she used to struggle with her weight. But when aerobics, leg warmers and workout routines for women became popular years ago, she was one of the first to get on board. She lost weight and found her passion: helping others reach their optimal fitness, a calling that has given her pleasure for nearly 30 years.

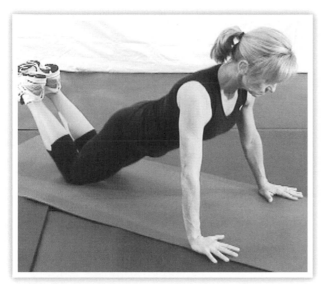

Diane started to teach 4•3•2•1—and went down a pants size.

You can imagine the excellent shape Diane was already in when she started to teach my 10-minute workouts. Although she did not lose any weight, she dropped 3% body fat and went down a pants size. People noticed that she looked thinner, and she herself noticed that she had greater endurance and stamina, and that it was easier to teach her fitness classes.

Having worked with people of all ages, Diane notes that it's never too late to start a fitness regimen. When people make poor choices or stop working out, she simply says, "The past is past. Every day you just restart, and re-commit." Diane says she loves helping people discover their inner athlete, and she particularly enjoys working with people who are stuck or need a boost. She says she feels like a proud parent when one of her clients discovers the benefits of personal fitness: "It feels good to know that you've helped someone out and you've made a difference."

Bill's Story:
Younger Each Year

Bill doesn't mind getting questions about his age, because his "body age" is that of a 30-year-old. He also doesn't mind attending reunions of his high school class of '69 because he seems to be getting younger while his classmates are all getting older.

A successful business entrepreneur with a driving energy level and a stimulating dash of ADD, Bill appears to live by the credo that things worth doing are worth doing at 150%. He's an example of what happens when you take 4•3•2•1 as far as you possibly can. He trains like a professional athlete, with a constant drive to improve. He also refuses to do at least two things. He refuses to let his belly hang over his belt, and he refuses to get old. His extraordinary commitment to personal fitness has enabled him to make good on both claims.

Before Bill discovered 4•3•2•1 through his wife, Sandy, he felt he was not getting the maximum benefit out of his long exercise sessions. He was tired during the day and even had to take naps, which affected his productivity and performance. He was frustrated, but not sure what to do differently. Today, he does multiple circuits of the 4•3•2•1 workouts and even adds extra core-strengthening exercises. Because of an old ankle injury, he can't do any running, but he can use a rowing machine and other equipment to stay in top form. Now he never naps, he needs less sleep at night, and he has an extraordinary endurance level that he hopes will allow him to keep doing the things he enjoys, like snowmobiling 200 miles into the wilderness, for many years to come. In fact, when a snowmobile accident threw

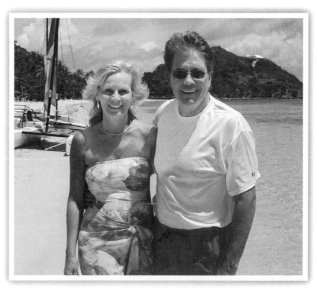

Bill (with wife Sandy) is a guy who simply refuses to get old.

him 60 feet through the air, his strength and stamina were probably what allowed him to walk away from the wreckage and drive home.

Bill is an example of what can be accomplished with total adherence to the 10-Minute Total Body Breakthrough. Today he is exercising less, he is stronger than ever, and he is experiencing more life. Formerly he was a respectable sedan. Now he's a race car.

And Now It's About You . . .

You, too, deserve a personal coach, and that"s what I aim to be. In this book, I'll show you exactly what you need to do to get into the best shape of your life and transform your future. I guarantee you will be not only happy with your physical changes, but also amazed by the effect your fitness will have on every-thing you do—and feel.

May I be the first to welcome you to the rest of your life.

Online 4•3•2•1 Support

To make sure you're successful with your 10-Minute Total Body Breakthrough program, check out the book's website at www.4321fitness.com. Here you'll find:

- 10-Minute coaching tips
- 10-Minute Challenge information and how to start your own "Take 10 to a New You" group
- Video clips that demonstrate specific 4•3•2•1 exercises.
- Original scientific articles and sources
- A place to upload your pictures and success stories

chapter 2

Fitness at the Speed of Life

Transformation in 10 Minutes a Day

To begin to be in the best shape of your life, you don't have to set your alarm clock earlier. You don't have to spend an hour and a half at the gym. You don't have to make time for exercising after a full day of work, when you finally drag yourself home and just want to relax. All you need to do is set aside 10 minutes—anytime, anywhere. You probably spend 10 minutes daydreaming about what you wish your life were like. Now you can use that time to make your dreams a reality.

Over and over again, I have seen my clients successfully meet their fitness goals. And they change more than just their waistlines. They gain greater energy, self-confidence and inner strength, which they use for an enormous range of personal dreams. You can be equally successful with your own quest to become the best possible *you*. Whether you prefer to do your fitness program in the privacy of your home, at a gym or with a group of friends or colleagues, I'll show you step by step how to reach your chosen goals.

How Busy Are You?

Do you carry over your "to do" list from one day to the next? Have some of the items on that list been there for weeks? Every day we try harder, do things faster, manage our time more efficiently and take our multitasking to new heights, yet we never seem to do enough.

Below are six reasons we are all busier than ever—so busy we feel that we can't stop to take care of our own health.

- **Many different roles.** These days we are no longer locked into gender stereotypes, so dads change diapers at home, moms go to the office, and both can enlist and go to war. The more roles we have—partner, parent, sibling, friend, coworker, committee chair, soccer coach, PTA member, church or temple volunteer, community organizer—the harder we have to work to do an acceptable job in each of them. Many of us are members of the "sandwich generation," meaning we take care of parents and children at the same time. Being in the middle brings obligations that can't be delegated to anyone else.

- **Overwork.** Companies are trying to get by with fewer employees, which increases the workload for everyone. Many of us bring work home from the office or work out of a home office, which blurs the line between "work" and "life." In the old days, we felt guilty about making personal calls during office hours. Now we take business calls during personal hours and don't think twice about it.

- **Information overload.** Headlines, breaking news, advertisements, phone calls, e-mail, instant messages and text messages vie for our attention all day long. If we step out of the information stream for a moment, we're immediately out of touch. If you're the kind of person who tries to stay on top of the news or to keep up with the latest developments in your field, you could spend the whole day just reading what's available in print and on the Internet.

- **Round-the-clock accessibility.** To "get away from it all," we have to go somewhere without cell phone reception. Good phone etiquette requires at best an immediate answer and at worst a callback within 24 hours. Bad phone etiquette is sending text messages from the dinner table or taking a call in the middle of a parent/teacher conference—but that doesn't stop people from doing it.

- **Instant obsolescence.** The minute you buy a computer—or a car, or a cell phone, or anything electronic—it becomes obsolete. If you are employee version 1.0, watch out for employee version 1.1 or, even worse, a company upgrade to employee 2.0. If you don't keep sharpening your skills, the next generation will take your place. We have to run as fast as we can just to stay put.

- **Unreasonable expectations.** We're all supposed to look fabulous and be rich and successful. We're expected to be brimming with self-confidence, charm and wit. Now that no one has any extra time, time-consuming activities are fashionable, like entertaining, decorating, baking cookies from scratch and creating homemade presents. Martha Stewart shows us how to serve perfect morning muffins to our houseguests—on four hours of sleep. All these endeavors take time, which is why celebrities have a small army of people who decorate their houses, buy their clothes, do their hair and makeup, and take care of their gift shopping for them.

When we try to meet all these obligations and to fulfill all our roles, we can end up making unsatisfying compromises, like showing up for the last half of our child's game or recital or letting someone else buy the gift while we sign the card. We are always thinking about several things at once, to the point where we are never 100% "present" for anyone. We pay the price for this pace of life in our relationships, as well as mentally, emotionally, spiritually . . . and, of course, physically.

10 Minutes Really *Can* Make a Difference

Most fitness gurus are still repeating the same old advice about the importance of 30 to 60 minutes of aerobic activity three to five times a week. You don't have that kind of time to spare—and now research shows you don't need it! Again, exercise does not have to be prolonged or painful to build muscles and give you a metabolic boost. As you'll learn in Chapter 4, short bursts of intense exercise are highly effective.

Even if you had enough time for all that cardiovascular exercise, your fitness regimen would not be complete without resistance training, core-strengthening exercises and stretching. People who focus on aerobic exercise—runners, for example—tend to overlook weight training. The reverse is also true: Weight lifters tend to ignore cardiovascular exercise and stretching. With my 4•3•2•1 program, you get a total body workout, including cardiovascular exercise, strengthening exercises, stretching and deep breathing, all crammed into 10 power-packed minutes. With each workout you will:

■ Boost your metabolism and energy level

■ Burn excess fat

■ Maintain and strengthen your muscles

■ Improve your flexibility and coordination

■ Maintain and build bone strength

■ Increase your endurance and stamina

■ Enhance your blood circulation

■ Improve your blood pressure and cholesterol levels

The Key to Fitness

The 4•3•2•1 system incorporates everything you need for a total body workout in just 10 minutes— an approach I call *fitness fusion.*

4 minutes of H.E.A.T.
(high-energy aerobic training)
+

3 minutes of resistance exercise
+

2 minutes of core-strengthening exercises
(abdominal, lower back and hip muscles)
+

1 minute of stretching and deep breathing

---

10 minutes of fitness fusion

The foregoing list of benefits is far from complete and doesn't even begin to address all the nonphysical changes you will experience as you become more and more fit. In my years as a fitness coach and personal trainer, I have learned that *motion affects emotion.* When you start taking better care of yourself, the rest of your life falls into place. With increased energy, strength, stamina and focus, you become less stressed and your relationships improve. Your productivity goes up. And eventually—just around the time other people begin to ask, *"What happened?"*—you become a role model, the person telling friends and family, "If I can do it, you can!"

Exercise for Everyone

Part of the beauty of this program is that it meets you at your current level, then takes you all the way to total fitness. I have worked with every kind of individual, from people with bad backs and sedentary office workers to aerobics instructors and elite athletes on national sports teams. Whether you haven't exercised since high school or you're already a fitness buff, this book is for you.

- **Beginner.** If you haven't exercised for a while or are not in especially good shape right now, you'll master one 10-minute workout at a time and gradually increase the difficulty of your sessions. If certain exercises are too challenging for you, just follow the tips I include for making them easier until you become stronger.

- **Intermediate.** Some of my most satisfied clients are people who exercised for years before discovering they can become *more fit* in *less time*. If you're already in reasonably good shape, the 10-minute workouts will be as challenging as you make them. Also, you can make your sessions more demanding by following my tips for increasing the difficulty of the exercises. In addition, if you have more than 10 minutes available, you can repeat certain sections of a 10-minute workout or repeat the entire circuit for an extra challenge.

- **Advanced.** If you're already a fitness buff, you may choose to focus on the most challenging variations of the exercises. If you have more than 10 minutes for exercising, you may wish to repeat certain sections of a 10-minute workout, and you also have the option of repeating the entire workout once or multiple times. I have trained elite athletes who do as many as six complete workouts in one session—and believe me, that's *hard*!

An example of this last approach is Pete. No stranger to difficult workouts, Pete used to be a professional athlete. "I had always been in shape," he says, "but after doing the 4•3•2•1 workouts I feel and look a lot leaner." Pete has noticed another benefit that he's excited about: "I feel my personality more. 'Who I am' is coming out more. Now I'm always animated. I have more enthusiasm. My attitude has changed tremendously. My wife definitely notices it!"

Three Levels + 12 Weeks = Total Body Fitness

The 4•3•2•1 program leads you from beginner to expert by showing you, step by step, how to progress through three levels of fitness:

- **Level I.** The workouts in Level I use only your bodyweight. No special equipment is necessary, and you don't have to belong to a gym.

- **Level II.** The workouts in Level II use inexpensive equipment, such as a jump rope, a flexible resistance band and an exercise ball.

- **Level III.** The workouts in Level III are designed for the use of professional equipment at the gym (or a home gym).

At each level, you will learn four different workouts, one per week. If you aren't sure how to do a reverse crunch, have no fear. You'll find detailed instructions, with pictures, for every exercise. By following the 28 days of daily instructions for each level, you'll know exactly what to do each day. This takes the guesswork out of getting fit and guarantees you will be successful. My clients tell me that these three months go very quickly. They're so encouraged by the positive feedback that the time flies by.

To get the full benefit of the program, I encourage everyone to start at Level I and move through all three levels. Some extremely fit individuals may find that Level I is not sufficiently challenging, but the vast majority of people will find that starting at the beginning works best. If you aren't sure what to do, your fitness assessment in Chapter 6 will show you where you should start.

Mixing It Up to Keep Boredom at Bay

You may dread spending your life on a treadmill at the gym, always looking at the same four walls. You may have watched the same exercise DVDs hundreds of times. Good news: The days of doing the same exercise routine again and again are over. This is important, because for most fitness regimens

One New Thing

Mixing up your exercise routines does more than keep you interested in working out each day. British psychologist Ben Fletcher discovered that when people try new things, they're more likely to lose weight. In his study, participants were asked to do one new thing every day. They were not required to focus on food or exercise, and they were not asked to use willpower to lose weight. They simply had to break their usual habits—and they lost an average of 11 pounds in four months by *not* thinking about weight loss!

burnout is a huge problem. People get tired of doing the same old thing and lose their motivation after a couple of months. Also, boredom can lead to carelessness while you're working out, which in turn can cause injury. I have built variety right into the 4•3•2•1 program in several ways:

- *In each 10-minute workout, you'll move quickly through many different exercises.* There's no time to get bored. Moving from one exercise to the next keeps you focused and ensures that you keep exercising at optimal intensity.

- *You can choose from 12 different 10-minute workouts.* Once you're familiar with all the exercises in all three levels, you can pick any of them to do on a particular day.

- *You can create your own challenging workouts.* After you learn how to do all the exercises, you can swap sections of different workouts. Since each of the 12 workouts has four sections, you can create hundreds of unique routines to suit your mood or circumstances. Just refer to the flip cards at the back of the book. No other exercise program gives you this kind of flexibility.

Even More Variety: Five Different Settings

You can do your 10-minute workouts anywhere. Little icons found on the flip cards tell you which locations are appropriate for each exercise.

Working out at home. If you're working out in the comfort of your own home, I'm assuming you can wear gym clothes and get down on the floor. Choose exercises with the "home" icon to put together a complete home workout using just your bodyweight or minimal equipment such as a jump rope, large exercise ball or flexible resistance band.

Working out outside. If it's a beautiful day, choose exercises with the "outdoors" icon and take your 4•3•2•1 workout outside. These workouts do not use gym equipment, although some use readily available props like steps or a park bench.

Working out at work. If you're stuck at the office, you can do a complete 10-minute workout at your desk by selecting exercises with the "work" icon. These workouts do not require you to put on gym clothes or to use exercise equipment. Ten minutes of exercising at your desk is more challenging than you might think—and it means you'll leave work more fit than you were when you arrived in the morning.

Working out while traveling. If you're on the road and looking for a workout to do in your hotel room, choose exercises with the "travel" icon. These workouts do not require large equipment and can be done almost anywhere.

Working out at the gym. If you belong to a gym (or have an advanced home gym), choose exercises with the "gym" icon. These require specialized equipment. I'll show you the best way to use gym equipment to get more muscle in minutes.

Being able to do the 10-minute workouts in a variety of settings is an important feature of the 4•3•2•1 program for many of my clients. Chip, who travels constantly, always throws his resistance bands into his suitcase. "I can do a workout in my hotel room," he says. "I could do one in the airport if I had to." He describes his experiences with characteristic humor: "The 4•3•2•1 exercise program is showing me that I have muscles in parts of my body that I haven't used since the Nixon administration!"

Making It Happen: How to Use This Book

Each chapter approaches your fitness program from a different angle. In Chapter 3, you'll determine your deepest motivation for getting fit. In Chapter 4, you'll find out why the program is not a gimmick, but a scientifically validated approach for fast fitness. Because healthy eating is an essential part of fitness, Chapter 5 presents the principles of "traffic light" eating and shows you how to use food as fuel for your body. In Chapter 6, you'll examine the barriers that formerly kept you from exercising and find out how to guarantee your success. Chapters 7, 8 and 9 contain four complete exercise routines for Levels I, II, and III. Each day you will also refer to Chapter 10, which includes three months' worth of specific daily instructions to help you reach your goal. And then, in Chapter 11, you'll learn about our corporate challenges and how to form your own Take 10 health and fitness group.

Read the book all the way to the end. You can skim Chapters 7, 8 and 9 because you'll be getting back to them when you start your fitness program. Once you're ready to begin, follow the daily instructions in Chapter 10 as you proceed through the three levels of fitness and learn all 12 of the 10-minute workouts.

Understanding the Daily Instructions

To ensure your success, I've included step-by-step guidelines for every day of the program. Each level has 28 days of daily instructions. You will learn a new workout once a week, for a total of four workouts at each level.

One of the reasons each level lasts 28 days is that conventional wisdom maintains it takes three to four weeks to create a new habit. We can't simply erase bad habits—they've been neurologically etched into our brains for years—but we can override them with healthier behavior. The first time you try a new, positive behavior, it makes fresh, exciting neurological connections in your brain. And the more you repeat it, the faster and more efficient this new mental "wiring" becomes.

Workouts That Beat Conventional Exercise

What are the advantages of the 4•3•2•1 workouts? Let me count the ways:

- They are doable. Anyone can do 10 minutes!
- They can be performed anywhere, anytime.
- They fit into anyone's schedule.
- They give maximum benefits in minimal time.
- They include every type of essential exercise, providing total body fitness.
- They can be adapted to any fitness level.
- They can be extended to any length of workout you want.
- They can be performed with or without equipment.
- They are never boring.

The daily instructions help you align your mind, body and soul with your new commitment to fitness. Every day has five components:

1. Move. To improve your health, there is no bigger step you can take than simply moving your body. Exercise transforms the way you think, feel, act and look. Ideally, you will perform your 4•3•2•1 workouts every other day (Monday, Wednesday and Friday, for example). On the days in between, you will keep up with your healthy lifestyle choices and do 10 minutes of cardiovascular exercise or some other physical activity that you enjoy. Possibilities include everything from jumping rope or jogging on the treadmill to playing basketball with the kids or kickboxing or tennis or swimming . . . well, you get the idea. The point is to keep moving!

2. Fuel. This section provides tips for healthy eating to supplement the general principles that are included in Chapter 5. Your goal is not to diet, but to establish new eating habits for life. No more counting calories, no more deprivation, no more unnecessary guilt, just tried-and-true strategies to help you reach your optimal weight and stay there.

3. Renew. In addition to exercise and food, your body needs rest and relaxation. This section provides tips for mental and physical rejuvenation, from getting a good night's sleep to stress management.

4. Connect. We are happiest and most successful when we're in touch with ourselves, our friends and family, our community and our faith. When we're connected to our goals and our sources of strength, we feel hopeful, empowered and supported. We make choices that are beneficial for ourselves and others. Every morning, I want you to ask yourself, "What do I want to change today?"; then "Why do I want to change?"; and finally "How can I move one inch closer?" Every evening, I want you to share your highs and lows with someone else. And before you go to bed, I want you to ask yourself, "What did I do well today?" This section has additional assignments that are designed to get you back in touch with the elements of your life that bring you strength.

Let me tell you a personal story that you might find useful. Every night at dinner my family plays a game called Highs and Lows. Each of us has an opportunity to share the best parts of our day (the highs) and to describe the most challenging parts

---

Taking Things Day by Day: How to Make It Happen

The 10-Minute Total Body Breakthrough program progresses through three fitness levels. This book contains not only all the workouts and exercise instructions you'll need, but also 28 days of step-by-step instructions for each level: 84 days in all (included in Chapter 10).

These daily instructions take the guesswork out of your new fitness regimen. As you follow the steps, you will become more fit. What's more, the instructions include special tips and tasks that help you maintain your enthusiasm, enrich your personal and spiritual life, and make sure you get all the support you need on this life-changing journey.

To give you an idea of how the daily instructions look, here are Day 1 and Day 28 from Level I. You may choose to jot a couple of notes in the book each day or create your own 10-Minute Total Body Breakthrough journal.

LEVEL I: Day 1

Move:

Today you will complete Level I, Workout 1 (page 103).

Fuel:

Buy some protein powder, and pick up some fruit and milk. Make your first 4•3•2•1 Protein Smoothie for breakfast or for a nutritious snack. (See pages 67–68 for recipes.)

Renew:

Get your beauty rest! A full, deep, restful sleep can help you de-stress after a long day and wake up refreshed, ready to begin again. While you sleep, you subconsciously process the events of the day. People often come up with solutions in the middle of the night—which is why, when you're in a quandary, people advise you to "sleep on it."

Connect:

If you could change one thing about yourself, what would it be? Imagine the best version of *you*. What would be different if you were as healthy and fit as you could possibly be? What would be different about your life? Who else would be affected by your transformation?

Journal:

_____

_____

_____

"What saves a man is to take a step. Then another step."

—*Antoine de Saint-Exupéry*

LEVEL I: Day 28

Move:

Today, take 10 minutes to do stretching movements while practicing your deep breathing. Give yourself a high-five. You have exercised every day for four weeks.

Fuel:

You've been drinking more water and improving your eating habits for four weeks. How do these changes make you feel? If you're an emotional eater, identify your triggers. Watch for any negative, self-defeating thoughts during the day. Write them down in your journal. (For more on stress and eating, see page 54.)

Renew:

Give yourself a "time out" today. Put a "Gone Renewing" sign on your door and don't let anyone disturb you.

Connect:

Text a love message. Whether it's to your spouse, a friend or a family member, send a cell phone message today and tell them how much you love or appreciate them.

Journal:

_____

_____

_____

"The measure of who we are is what we do with what we have."

—*Vince Lombardi*

(the lows). This always makes for lively family discussions. More important, it provides us with some precious time for caring for and supporting one another. I have found that even when we're rushed, just a few minutes of conversation—sharing our hearts, our highs and lows—leaves us feeling stronger and more closely connected.

I'll be asking you to do the same kind of sharing every day with your family or with a friend you trust. If you live alone, you might save up your experiences and share them with someone at week's end. You'll be amazed at the difference this makes in your physical and emotional health.

5. Journal. If you already keep a journal, you know how valuable it is to record your thoughts and feelings about each day's events. In order to put down something meaningful and articulate, you have to first shape your ideas and make sense of your experiences. Sometimes the act of writing will reveal the hidden significance of a thought or event, or remind you of something you might otherwise have overlooked. In addition, it's important to write down your goals. Every day, you have the opportunity to take one step closer to achieving what you want. This is your chance to write down what you hope to attain and to determine the steps that will help you get there. I encourage you to write about your progress and at the very least make a note of your successes so you can build on them the next day.

The Flip Cards

After you've completed all three levels of the program, use the flip cards at the back of the book to vary your exercise sessions. I've broken down each workout into its four separate sections and put all the sections on separate cards. You'll be able to mix-and-match sections from different workouts to create hundreds of new exercise routines. No other exercise program has ever provided this kind of flexibility! If, at any time, you need to refresh your memory about a particular exercise, just refer to the pages on which it is fully described. As you can tell from the special binding and the flip cards, this book is designed to be used repeatedly as a reference. You will want to keep it handy, not sitting on a bookshelf.

Discovering Your Inner Athlete

When it comes to starting a fitness program, many people feel intimidated. They look at the super-toned bodies in magazines, on television and at the gym, and they think exercising is only for the Beautiful People. Well, you don't have to be perfect to be fit, so stop worrying about what other people look like and remember that *time is passing*. You can sit on the sidelines and think about becoming fit . . . or you can take action and make a little bit of progress every day. Days will turn into weeks, and weeks will turn into months, and one day you'll realize that little by little you have made tremendous changes.

The 4•3•2•1 workouts will make you feel so much better that you'll feel bad when you miss them. Before long, you'll be exercising not because you *ought* to but because you *want* to. And as you become stronger, you'll find other ways to add more activity to your normal day. No more driving around in circles looking for a parking space close to the store. No more waiting for the elevator when you can take the stairs. You'll be getting together with friends for walking dates instead of dinner dates. You'll have the energy to take a long bike ride or play outside with your kids. You'll have the stamina for a lengthy visit to the museum or even a walking tour abroad.

I believe there is an inner athlete in all of us. One of the reasons I love my job is that over and over again I get to see people discover—or rediscover—their inner drive to be healthy and fit. This desire is like a star that burns inside each of us. Sometimes it nearly goes out or is obscured by illness or misfortune, but never doubt that it's there, waiting to shine brightly into every part of your life.

chapter 3

What Is Your "Why"?

Finding Your Motivation to Change

Let's say you open your newspaper one morning and there's a front-page story: MAGIC PILL INTRODUCED. Good news! Scientists have designed a miracle medication that will lower your risk of diabetes, obesity, heart disease, stroke and several types of cancer. This medication will also rev up your metabolism, help you burn body fat and give you more energy. In addition, it will strengthen and tone your muscles, maintain your bone strength, reduce anxiety and depression, ward off Alzheimer's disease, help you look years younger and improve your sex life. What's more, this magic pill has few side effects, it's cheap and it's available everywhere! You would run out and get it, right?

Of course, the magic pill is actually exercise, and you can take advantage of it right now. The physical benefits of exercise are extensive and well documented, as are the effects of exercise on mood and stress. And thanks to the 4•3•2•1 program, we now know that getting fit can change your life.

Over the years, as we tested the 4•3•2•1 workouts, we began to see interesting side effects. People not only increased their regular exercise, but also were more likely to make other important changes in their lives. Reports of greater self-esteem, more self-control, increased happiness, improved lifestyle, better relationships and spiritual enhancement all poured in.

Moving your body on a regular basis transforms your life because *success creates success*. Exercise—even just a little bit—changes everything. Not just the way you look and feel, but also the way you think and, ultimately, the way you live your life.

My intention is to get you moving right away. Sometimes a short-term goal is all that's needed to get going, but putting a picture of yourself in a bathing suit on the refrigerator goes only so far. Besides, we all have a tendency to let ourselves off the hook when we're seriously tempted, or when we feel rushed, tired or sad. By finding a worthy goal, it's easier for us to hold ourselves to the highest standard.

What Goals Do You Want to Achieve?

What are your truest aspirations—your deepest desires and highest ambitions? Do you want to start a business, have a baby, cook the perfect pie crust, learn to play the accordion, build a retirement home, go to Venice or travel into space? What are you already doing now that a new you could do better? Maybe your highest priority is to stay right where you are but grow your business, focus on your marriage or become a better parent.

My personal philosophy, shaped by years of playing on the football field, is that anything that's worth doing is worth doing well. But when you have no energy and are feeling fatigued, you can't expect to perform at a level that will bring you the success you desire. Whatever your goals are, you'll need strength and stamina to achieve them.

Visualize Your Success

Throughout the ages, people of almost every culture have believed in the power of thought. Some people believe that our thoughts literally determine our destiny; others simply believe in the power of positive thinking. It is well known in the field of sports psychology that Olympic athletes mentally rehearse each of their routines, whether it's a difficult maneuver on the parallel bars or skiing the slalom on an icy course requiring split-second timing, and that vividly imagining their success enhances their performance. Thoughts are powerful . . . so let's put yours to work for you.

First, imagine what will happen if you keep going the way you are now, without making any changes in your lifestyle. What kind of shape will you be in next year? In another five years? Will you be able to accomplish everything you would like to do in your life, or will you need to make some sacrifices because of your health?

Now take a moment to imagine yourself fit and strong. If you can go back in time and remember a period when you were healthy and energetic, recall what it felt like to be full of strength and vitality. Your body holds that memory in its cells. If going backward doesn't work for you, then go forward and picture yourself as fit as you can possibly be. What does your face look like? How about your body? Are you slimmer, stronger, more toned? Do you look younger, prettier, more handsome? How do you feel about yourself? Are you happier, more confident, more hopeful? What's different about your personal relationships?

What Are Your Dreams?

When you have the kind of body you look forward to and the energy you need every day, how will you be a better partner, parent, friend, relative, coworker or volunteer? How will these changes affect your career, your spirituality and the quality of your life? What will you be able to do better? In what ways could you be more successful, productive and fulfilled? What could you accomplish with your renewed stamina and enthusiasm? What strands from your life would you like to go back and pick up again? What might you try for the first time?

Once you become the best possible version of *you*, you'll have the strength and energy to experience *more life*. As you maximize your fitness, you'll also be maximizing your contribution to the world: improving your relationships, increasing your productivity at work and becoming a better spouse, parent, friend, relative and colleague. With more agility and resilience, you'll even have more fun when you're relaxing. When my work is getting to me, I'm likely to call a "board meeting"—a boogie board meeting, that is!

Check those benefits of exercise that might inspire you to meet your goals.

☐ **Exercise keeps you physically fit.** It produces a capable body that is strong, straight and flexible.

☐ **Exercise combats fatigue and boosts energy.** It increases your stamina and endurance, making it easier to accomplish everyday tasks and to achieve long-term goals.

☐ **Exercise prepares a woman's body for pregnancy, delivery and postpartum recovery.** Also, moderate weight-bearing exercise three to five times per week produces babies who are larger and heavier. (If you're pregnant, consult your doctor before beginning any exercise program.)

Are You Unhappy with Your Weight or Appearance?

If you're currently dissatisfied with your weight or appearance, don't be discouraged. You are a work in progress—a masterpiece waiting to be unveiled. Keep your focus on the trim, healthy body that will emerge along the way, and remember that each small step in a positive direction—doing a few minutes of exercise, for example, or making one small change in eating habits—places you on the right path.

Keep in mind that the numbers on your bathroom scale do not indicate how fit you are. Some thin people may be very weak and unhealthy, while some heavier individuals who exercise regularly may actually be in good shape. If your weight stays the same but you change your body composition by decreasing fat and increasing muscle, then you have become more fit. You will look and feel better, and your clothes will fit better, even though you haven't lost weight.

Check the benefits that will help you improve your weight or appearance.

☐ **Exercise burns excess body fat.** Combined with sensible eating, exercise helps you lose weight.

☐ **Exercise gives you a metabolic boost.** After an intense 10-minute workout, your metabolism will remain elevated for several hours. This means you'll be burning extra calories whether you're actively going about your day or sleeping. The harder you work during your exercise session, the greater the metabolic boost will be and the more calories you'll burn afterward.

☐ **Exercise builds muscles, which in turn burn more calories.** A pound of fat burns two calories per day, while a pound of muscle burns six calories per day. This may not sound like much—but it's an increase of 300%! When you follow the 10-Minute Total Body Breakthrough program, your new muscle-added body will burn more calories, even at rest, than your old body.

☐ **Exercise keeps you handsome/beautiful.** By boosting the circulation to your skin and scalp, exercise helps keep your complexion clear and your hair healthy.

Are You Getting Older?

Too many of us assume we're "getting old" when we hit a certain age and find it harder to do things—harder to get out of bed in the morning, harder to run upstairs, harder to bend over and tie shoelaces. But having a few more birthdays does not mean you must be less fit. I encourage you to question your assumptions about "getting old," because you may be settling for aches and pains instead of reaching for strength and flexibility. It is absolutely possible to stay physically fit well into old age. One of my favorite pictures—you may have seen it—is of a silver-haired grandmother in a wet suit, standing next to her surfboard. Doesn't that say it all?

I like to tell people there are two ages: chronological age and "body age." Your chronological age is based on the date you were born, whereas your body age is determined by your physical health and fitness, including your cardiovascular endurance, bone density, muscle strength, flexibility, blood pressure, blood chemistry and percentage of body fat. I have tested individuals in their twenties who were physically as old as individuals in their fifties. But I also have clients in their seventies whose body ages are in their thirties or forties. You can turn back your body's clock so you look and feel 10, 20 or 30 years younger.

Exercise can help reverse age-related changes in your body. Check those benefits that apply to you.

☐ **Exercise fights sarcopenia, the loss of muscle that naturally occurs with age.** It also helps to improve balance, coordination and agility, which can reduce the risk of falls later in life.

☐ **Exercise helps to relieve the symptoms of menopause.** These may include hot flashes, mood swings and sleep problems.

☐ **Exercise combats osteoporosis.** In the five to seven years following menopause, women can lose up to a fifth of their bone mass. However, thinning bones are a health concern for women of any age. Weight-bearing exercise helps to keep bones strong.

Exercise Has Been Shown to Decrease the Risk of Dementia

In 1967, 100 sets of Swedish twins were enrolled in a study called HARMONY. Thirty years later, researchers tried to determine why, in 90 cases, one twin developed dementia while the other did not. Since each set of twins was genetically identical, this presented a unique opportunity to study the effects of lifestyle choices and environmental factors on age-related mental decline. The study concluded that light exercise, such as gardening or walking, and regular exercise involving sports were associated with a reduced risk of dementia. Higher levels of exercise seem to be associated with an even lower risk of dementia.

Are You Interested in Keeping Your Brain Sharp?

An ever-growing body of research indicates that physical activity is beneficial for your brain. Learning to do new things—trying unfamiliar exercises, for example—promotes new neural pathways in your brain, so it's good to vary your routines every day. Mix it up by brushing your teeth with the other hand, holding the phone to the other ear, taking a different route to work or standing on one foot while you do the dishes.

Studies suggest that the more you exercise, the more your brain will benefit from it, especially considering "executive" functions such as planning, organization, working memory and inhibiting inappropriate behavior—abilities that tend to decline as we get older. Of particular relevance here is the finding that exercise programs using both aerobic exercise and strength training produce better results for cognitive abilities than either type of exercise done by itself.

Scientists have also discovered that physically fit people experience less shrinkage of the frontal cortex of their brain with age. If you have a family history of Alzheimer's disease, you'll be interested to hear that exercise decreases the risk of dementia.Laboratory studies indicate that exercise is associated with actual

Rachel's Checkup
Facing the Reality (and Myths) of Getting Older

A lot of "getting old" is due to a vicious cycle that starts with losing muscle mass. To illustrate the usual context of advancing age, let's take a look at Rachel, a mother of three who is now 50 years old.

Rachel has been a nurse all her adult life. She gained a few pounds with each pregnancy, plus a few more pounds when she hit menopause. In addition, she has experienced an age-related loss of muscle mass. At the end of her workday, Rachel is so tired that she barely has enough energy to cook dinner when she gets home. She laughs and says it's because she's "as old as dirt." Actually, Rachel is exhausted because she's caught in

a vicious cycle. And if she doesn't do something to break the cycle, she can expect to become even weaker and more vulnerable to illness and injury.

Starting around the age of 45, most people begin to lose muscle tissue at the rate of about 0.5% to 1% per year—a process known as sarcopenia. Losing muscle makes it more difficult to do things, so we become less active and lose more muscle, which makes it harder to be active. At the same time, the less we do, the less energy we have to do more. In addition, when muscle mass declines, metabolism decreases along with it—as much as 5% every 10 years. If we continue to eat the same way as we age, we end up

gaining weight. We get softer, and parts of us begin to "go south."

For all these reasons, Rachel's doctor has encouraged her to start working out. He emphasized that a decline in metabolism is *not* a necessary part of aging—that it does *not* happen to women who get regular endurance exercise. He also advised her that exercise would reduce her risk for osteoporosis. When he recommended that she exercise for at least 30 minutes five days a week, Rachel nodded and smiled, but inside she was thinking, *You don't have the slightest idea what my life is like, do you?*

And that's where the 4•3•2•1 program comes in.

physical changes in the brain, including an increase in the number of large-diameter cerebral blood vessels and an increase in blood flow in the three major cerebral arteries. Exercise has also been shown to promote new cell growth in the brain.

Exercise has been shown to improve mental clarity. Do these benefits interest you?

☐ **Exercise can enhance your cognitive abilities.** Research shows that physical exercise at any age, especially when aerobic and resistance training are combined, has a beneficial effect on brain function.

☐ **Exercise reduces the risk of developing Alzheimer's disease.** An article in *The New York Times* entitled "Exercise on the Brain," by Sandra Aamodt and Sam Wang, notes that individuals who get regular exercise in middle age are one-third as likely to develop Alzheimer's disease in their seventies as those who do not exercise. Even people who don't start exercising until their sixties have their risk cut in half.

Is Your Life Filled with Too Much Stress?

When you're under stress, your body releases hormones such as adrenaline and cortisol. Adrenaline increases the heart rate, elevates blood pressure and makes energy available for "fight or flight." Cortisol increases blood sugar levels and enhances the brain's use of glucose; it also suppresses bodily activities such as digestion, reproduction and growth.

The activation of these hormones is critical if you're being physically attacked, but it serves no purpose in times of mental or emotional stress. Increased responsibilities at work, taking care of a sick child, falling behind on the bills or other causes of chronic stress can produce elevated levels of cortisol for months or years. Situations that can stress the body and elevate cortisol levels include illness, trauma, exposure to toxins, severe calorie restriction, physical exertion, excessive exercising, dehydration, sleep deprivation or drinking large amounts of alcohol.

Physical Problems Associated with Chronic Stress

When you have elevated levels of stress hormones over a long period of time, your mental and emotional stress will begin to manifest itself in physical problems, such as those listed below.

- Loss of muscle mass
- Elevated heart rate
- Suppressed immune function
- Obesity; abdominal fat

- High blood pressure
- High cholesterol
- Heart disease
- Increased blood sugar; diabetes

- Suppressed thyroid function
- Digestive problems; ulcers
- Bone loss; decrease in bone density
- Infertility

Our bodies need some cortisol in order to function correctly, but high levels of this hormone are associated with all kinds of serious physical problems. One such problem is loss of muscle tissue, which leads to a loss of strength, which in turn leads to inactivity, lowered metabolism, weight gain and ultimately problems like obesity and heart disease. Trust me, you do *not* want to go down that road. And you don't have to.

Learning to cope with stress constructively is an essential step toward having a healthy body. By exercising just 10 minutes a day, you can ease your stress and bring down your cortisol levels. In addition, when you take advantage of other readily available stress relievers such as social support, relaxation techniques and good nutrition, the payoff includes peace of mind, improved health and most likely a longer, happier life. The 10-Minute Total Body Breakthrough program will teach you how to work these stress management strategies into your busy lifestyle every day of the week.

Exercise can help to ease the strain of everyday living.

☐ **Exercise relieves stress.** After exercising, you feel more relaxed and less anxious. Bringing down your levels of stress hormones such as cortisol can have a big impact on your overall health.

☐ **Exercise helps you sleep.** Research shows that regular cardiovascular exercise can help you beat insomnia and eliminate the need for medication to help you sleep.

Are You Troubled by Depression?

Would you rather take an antidepressant or do some exercises? This is not just an idle question. Many people report that exercise lifts their mood. Some report that they feel a "runner's high" after intense exercise. Research has shown that exercise can be as effective as medication in relieving the symptoms of major depression.

You don't have to have major depressive disorder to feel bad. Many people who are somewhat depressed try to make themselves feel better, consciously or unconsciously, with food, recreational drugs or alcohol, but in the long run self-medication doesn't solve the underlying problem, and it also carries health risks. A 10-minute workout will improve your mood *and* leave you healthier.

Exercise Can Relieve Depression in People over 50

A study by James A. Blumenthal and a team of researchers at Duke University Medical Center took 156 patients between the ages of 50 and 77 who had been diagnosed with major depressive disorder (MDD) and randomly assigned them to three groups: exercise, medication (antidepressants) and a combination of exercise and medication. The patients in the exercise group spent 30 minutes riding a stationary bicycle, walking or jogging three times a week. The patients receiving medication showed a faster initial response, but after 16 weeks all three groups showed statistically significant and identical improvement in standard measurements of depression.

Do you want to improve your mood?

□ **Exercise has its own antidepressant value.** Over the long term, regular exercise can influence your mood as effectively as an antidepressant.

□ **Exercise relieves depression.** In the short term, exercise can lift your mood.

Do You Have Ongoing Health Issues or a Family History of Disease?

The fact is, if you're experiencing just about any problem with your health, the 10-Minute Total Body Breakthrough program will help you be as fit as you possibly can. Moreover, if you have a bad back, a trick knee or arthritis in your wrists, you can still use the 10-minute workouts to build your strength and resilience. In many cases, consistent exercise helps to make movements less painful. If you have a chronic illness like fibromyalgia, or if you're living with cancer, moderate exercise can help boost your health and stamina.

If cardiovascular health is an issue, please know that I have hundreds of clients who successfully lowered their cholesterol and blood pressure levels to the point at which they could throw away their medications.

Many of my clients have an oh-no moment when they first realize they're on the same path as family members who suffered from cardiovascular disease, diabetes or cancer. But knowledge is power. If you know you have a genetic predisposition to a certain illness, you can take steps to reduce your risk. Regular exercise is one of these steps. For example, you can counter the risk of cardiovascular problems by exercising regularly along with making healthy food choices. By helping to control blood sugar levels and weight, regular exercise is also effective in reducing the risk of diabetes. In addition, research has shown that people who exercise are less likely to become cancer patients than those who maintain a sedentary lifestyle.

Which benefit(s) below would improve your health or help you fight a genetic predisposition to illness?

□ **Exercise boosts cardiovascular fitness.** It will lower your heart rate, keep your heart pumping blood more efficiently and help control your blood pressure. If you also make the right food choices and stop smoking, you'll eliminate the three greatest risk factors for heart attack or stroke: sedentary lifestyle, unhealthy diet and tobacco.

□ **Exercise affects cholesterol levels.** It actually changes your blood chemistry, bringing down the "bad" cholesterol and raising the "good" cholesterol. It also brings down your serum triglycerides.

□ **Exercise boosts your immune system.** Moderate exercise boosts immunity, helps to speed wound healing in older adults and can be beneficial for patients undergoing treatment for cancer.

□ **Exercise improves mobility and reduces pain.** Joint or back pain can be relieved by regular exercise.

□ **Exercise lowers the risk of diabetes.** Regular exercise is associated with a drop in insulin resistance (a precursor of diabetes) and according to the American Diabetes Association is more effective than medication in delaying the development of type 2 diabetes.

□ **Exercise reduces the risk of certain cancers.** Activity reduces the risk of colon cancer and breast cancer, and it appears to protect against other types of cancer as well.

□ **Exercise improves your sex life.** Exercise enhances sexual functioning. Men who are obese and inactive are 2.5 times more likely to have erectile dysfunction.

□ **Exercise corrects constipation.** Don't laugh! Many people take over-the-counter preparations for this problem, when walking around the block would most likely be just as effective.

The "Why" Behind Your "Why": Your Deepest Motivation

Remember that child inside you who used to keep asking questions until there were no more to be asked? It's time to bring that child out again. Whenever you come up with a reason for exercising, ask yourself: "Why is that important?" This process will get you to the heart of the matter and let you discover your most powerful motivation.

It is not unusual for people to start exercising for one reason and then discover another reason as they get going. I remember when Denice started the 4•3•2•1 program after trying unsuccessfully for years to lose weight and get in shape. This time she took a different approach. Denice explains: "These grandkids came along, and I thought, 'I want to be around for them. I want to play with them. *I want to be a fit grandmother!*'" She resolved to exercise and eat healthy foods, and thinking about her grandchildren helped her reach her goals. Denice is stronger, healthier and more energetic today then she was 25 years ago. And most important, she is actively enjoying every day with her grandkids.

When you look for the "why" *behind* your "why," you will see that the most lasting motivation comes from your heart. We all want to love and be loved, to understand and be understood. We want the best for those we care about, and we look for the support that will bring out the best in ourselves.

Finding Your Most Powerful Motivation

Ask yourself these questions:

- What one thing is at the center of my life?
- Why do I get up in the morning?
- What is it that motivates me to be healthy and to live well?

Are We Too Busy for Our Own Good?

We're all working so hard and running so fast that many of us have become disconnected from ourselves, our loved ones, our community, our faith. We put our dreams and relationships on hold and focus on just getting by. We forget how to be self-nurturing. We start picking up bad habits and settling for second best. We may take a job we don't like, choose a partner who is less than ideal or follow someone who is giving us bad advice.

The farther away we get from our true hopes and aspirations, the more likely we are to start overdoing. We're busy, busy, busy—but not happy! We may try to numb ourselves to disappointments with too much television or alcohol or drugs. We start feeling negative emotions and get into negative thinking. Instead of having an inner coach who says, "Go for it! You can do it!" we develop an inner critic who says, "Don't bother. You'll never succeed." The end result is that we don't have enough energy to overcome the barriers that keep us from starting a fitness program.

If You Want to Help Others, Help Yourself

We've all heard a flight attendant give the instructions about flying with children. In the event of an emergency, the oxygen masks will drop down and you should immediately take one and put it on . . . your own face. If you're a parent, this advice is counterintuitive. The first person you want to protect is your child. However, you won't be able to help your child if you're out of the picture, so the first priority is to take care of yourself.

The same holds true for the rest of your life. To take care of others effectively, you need to be strong and rested. Your contribution is important to the lives and destinies of many others. But when you're tired, out of shape, irritable, impatient, anxious and stressed, you're in no shape to support others. Physically, you're limited in how much you can do. Mentally, you can't think straight or make good decisions. Emotionally, the well is dry. Spiritually, you feel empty instead of full.

The most important part of any juggling act is not the balls, or knives, or flaming torches, but the juggler. When you're juggling multiple roles and responsibilities, you need to stay strong. It is not "selfish" to get the exercise, rest, relaxation and nutrition you need to stay in top shape. To be the best possible version of yourself, you need abundant energy and endurance, mental clarity, physical strength, emotional resilience and spiritual contentment. When you're in top form, you'll be more attentive as a partner, more patient and loving as a parent, more loyal as a friend, more productive and successful at work, more diligent as a community volunteer and better able to handle the challenges of taking care of aging parents.

Another benefit of radiant health is feeling empowered and resilient rather than vulnerable and victimized. I remember working with a client who had recently undergone bypass surgery. He had dedicated every waking minute to becoming a successful entrepreneur, until one day he had a heart attack and nearly died. "Sean," he said, "if I attain all my business goals but lose my health in the process . . . how is that helping my family?" Because of his brush with death, he realized his true desire is to take care of his family—which means taking care of himself. Today, he has more energy, greater stamina and more zest for life than he's had in years. And his business is more successful than ever!

The greatest asset you bring to your family, your business or your mission is *you*. Your passion, your energy, your concern. Make yourself the top priority for just 10 minutes a day. Invest these few minutes in yourself and you'll be able to accomplish your life goals and enrich the lives of everyone around you.

Below are some reasons other people have given for making a commitment to personal fitness. Which reason applies to you, too?

☐ "I'm middle-aged, but I have two young daughters and I want to be able to dance with them at their weddings."

☐ "When I get home from work, I'm tired and cranky and my kids look for ways to stay away from me. I want to turn that around."

☐ "I want to be able to play with my grandchildren!"

☐ "My father died of a heart attack when I was 10 years old. I don't want that to happen to me— or to my kids."

☐ "I want to be my son's hero."

☐ "Others are counting on me. I need to be in top shape in order to take care of them."

☐ "As a single parent, everything depends on me. I can't afford to get sick."

The Importance of Feeling Connected

So what's the best way to start thinking about our own best interests? How do we get to the point where we're eating the right foods, exercising regularly and choosing healthy habits? By connecting to our personal and spiritual strengths and by reinforcing our most meaningful relationships.

When we connect, something profound happens. We feel full. We have hope. We have faith. We experience strength, recognizing power that we didn't know

---

Finding Your Sources of Strength

Ask yourself these questions:

• What or who brings strength and power into my life?

• What or who helps me overcome difficulties?

• What or who brings me vitality and endurance?

• Where can I go to get hope, meaning and purpose for my life?

• How often do I connect to the sources that provide me with the energy I will need if I am to be my very best?

was available. And when we feel strong, we begin to naturally choose the things we know are best for us. One person who came a very long way is Linda, who lost interest in her appearance after her husband died. She hated the way she looked in the mirror, so she just stopped looking. She knew she wanted to lose a little weight, so she tried the 10-minute workouts. Within a few short weeks, she felt so much better that she started exercising in earnest. Eventually, looking for ways to socialize that did not focus on food, she started calling friends for walking dates and even invited a group of friends over to learn how to hula dance. Linda notes, "I feel stronger as a human being—spiritually, mentally and physically. I'm just thrilled."

In fact, reliable research has shown that feeling connected—experiencing love, acceptance, support and nurturing—can have tremendous health benefits. Referring to religious involvement (regularly attending a place of worship, such as a church, temple or mosque), Harold G. Koenig, M.D., of Duke University, reported in the *Journal of the American Medical Association* that "the magnitude of the possible impact on physical health—particularly survival—may approximate that of abstaining from cigarette smoking or adding 7 to 14 years of life."

No matter what your religious beliefs may be, making a commitment to being the best possible *you* will allow you to nurture yourself again, develop positive relationships and heal your spirit. With renewed strength and confidence, you will reconnect with the values, people and activities that make your life positive, passionate, adventurous, loving, joyful and fun.

chapter 4

The Science Behind 4·3·2·1

Learn the Secrets to Your Success

The big event was coming up. The Class of 1984 from Amber Ridge High School was having its 25th reunion, and twin sisters Jill and Laura were looking at the pictures in their yearbook, each lost in her own thoughts. Finally, Jill broke the silence. "Did we really look that good?" she asked. "What if nobody recognizes us when we get there?"

"Don't be silly," Laura said. "Besides, everybody else will have changed just as much as we have." She paused and then added: "Except for Debbie Meyers. I bet she's still a size zero!"

The sisters looked at each other in dismay. "Is there enough time for the South Beach?" Jill whispered. "Or maybe the gym?"

"Oh, please!" exclaimed Laura. "Do you really want to go back to eating frozen raisins one at a time? And forget the gym! With a full-time job and three kids to worry about, I'm lucky if I can squeeze a shower into my schedule. Isn't there any kind of program that will fit into my life?"

Fitness Fusion– and How It Works

As it turned out, Jill went back to the treadmills at the gym, while Laura made an appointment with me to discuss the 10-Minute Total Body Breakthrough. Like everyone else who first hears about my program, Laura was wondering how 10 minutes could make a real difference. I told her that "more" is not necessarily "better" when it comes to exercise and that I had cut through mountains of scientific research to put together a fast-paced workout that she could fit into her hectic schedule. To explain my approach to fitness fusion, I outlined the different kinds of exercise that make each 10-minute workout so effective.

Circuit Training

Back in the '50s, researchers R.E. Morgan and G.T. Anderson at the University of Leeds in England developed *circuit training*, in which different exercises are performed one after the other, with little or no rest in between. (The name is based on the concept of an electrical circuit.) Over the years, circuit training has been used extensively in military and athletic arenas. It has finally gone mainstream because people are discovering that shorter, higher-intensity workouts yield greater results. Circuit training burns more calories than conventional cardiovascular exercise, and it increases muscular tone and definition.

In my 10-minute workout, you move quickly from one exercise to the next. This contributes to the effectiveness of the exercise. A complete 4•3•2•1 workout is considered one circuit.

Interval Training

Another essential element of each 4•3•2•1 workout is *high-intensity interval training*. This part of the workout includes cardiovascular exercise to elevate your heart rate, but with a twist: You raise and then lower the intensity of your exercise, a technique also known as "burst" training. I call it H.E.A.T., which stands for high-energy aerobic training. The H.E.A.T. approach is to alternate 30 seconds of moving as fast as you can with 30 seconds of exercising at a moder-

ate pace. Each 30-second interval of intense activity raises your heart rate and makes you sweat. During these periods, you exercise as hard as you can without losing your form. During the 30-second intervals of moderate activity, you recover and catch your breath. Alternating between fast and slow allows you to push much harder than you would if you tried only to sustain "fast" activity. The fast/slow approach is easier to handle, both physically and mentally.

Resistance Training

Strengthening exercises are forms of *resistance training,* so called because your body is given something to work against. This could be your own bodyweight, light equipment like a resistance band or weighted equipment at the gym.

Most popular resistance training programs were modeled after bodybuilding regimens with the primary goal of increasing the size, strength or definition of an isolated muscle or muscle group. For the purposes of general fitness, isolated muscle training has several drawbacks. It limits the number of muscles recruited and trained per exercise; it requires 8 to 12 exercises per workout, which usually takes up to an hour per session to complete; and it does not maximize the number of calories burned.

For my 4•3•2•1 workouts, I chose exercises that activate the large muscle groups (chest, shoulders, core, back, legs) and the smaller assisting muscles (biceps, forearm, triceps, calf) at the same time. These *compound resistance exercises* provide a safer, faster, more intense and more effective approach than isolated muscle training. They're also metabolism boosters, because the large muscle groups recruit significant energy; by training them, you increase the total amount of calories you expend during a workout. And they're time-efficient. You can train two or three muscle groups in one movement, so you get the greatest return for your investment of time.

Several routines in each 4•3•2•1 workout combine compound resistance exercises with *functional exercises*. Functional exercises are those that strengthen the muscles we typically use every day when we push, pull, lift, twist, squat down or reach up.

Putting It All Together

Each 4•3•2•1 workout packs every type of beneficial exercise into one 10-minute session. This means you'll be performing circuit training, high-intensity interval training and compound/functional resistance exercises, as well as exercises to strengthen your core followed by stretching and deep breathing. When done together, all these exercises provide you with a power-packed workout that maximizes your metabolism and fitness. There are many competing fitness programs available, but I am not aware of any other 10-minute program that combines all of these different types of important exercises into *one session*. With the fitness fusion of 4•3•2•1, you complete just one circuit to rev up your metabolism, tone and firm your muscles, and burn excess body fat—all in just 10 minutes.

④ minutes of H.E.A.T

Every workout starts out with 4 minutes of H.E.A.T. (high-energy aerobic training). I have included different kinds of cardiovascular activities in different workouts. You can choose to march in place, jump rope, jog on the treadmill or use a stair-climber, stationary bicycle or rowing machine—whatever you feel like doing!

Because you alternate high-intensity activity with a period of moderate activity, your H.E.A.T. cardiovascular workout goes like this:

    30 seconds of moderate activity
+ 30 seconds of high-intensity activity
+ 30 seconds of moderate activity
+ 30 seconds of high-intensity activity
+ 30 seconds of moderate activity
+ 30 seconds of high-intensity activity
+ Final 30 seconds of moderate activity—
   catch your breath, one more to go!
+ Final 30 seconds of H.E.A.T.—
   challenge yourself!

= Grand total: ④ minutes

After completing your 4 minutes of H.E.A.T., you continue directly to the next part of the workout without resting.

Boost Your Metabolism and Burn More Calories

After you work out, your body continues to need oxygen at a higher rate than it did before you started. This "after-burn"—that is, the calories expended after exercise—is referred to as EPOC (excess post-exercise oxygen consumption). EPOC is the rate of oxygen consumption above resting level that your body uses to return to its pre-exercise state. This is one of the great benefits of exercise, although few people know about it.

It can take up to 48 hours for your body to fully recover after a workout, depending on the intensity and duration of your exercise. Most of the fat burn associated with high-intensity workouts occurs *after* exercising, not during the workout itself. Your body will burn more calories long into the day and even while you're sleeping!

As you might expect, there is a relationship between the intensity of your exercise and how much your metabolism is elevated. As intensity increases, so do the magnitude and duration of EPOC. Multiple studies have shown that short, intense workouts burn more calories than longer periods of moderate exercise.

H.E.A.T. Produces Greater Energy Expenditure than Conventional Exercise

In a study at the University of New South Wales and the Garvan Institute, 45 overweight women were randomly assigned to two groups. Both groups exercised three times a week on stationary bikes. The women in Group A exercised for 20 minutes, alternating between 8 seconds of high-intensity activity and 12 seconds of moderate-intensity activity. The women in Group B exercised for 40 minutes—twice as long—at a continuous, regular pace. The members of Group A lost *three times* more weight. Researchers concluded that short bursts of activity with short rest periods produce greater energy expenditure than long periods of work and rest.

Lose More Body Fat

Many fitness buffs are concerned about the number of calories they burn during a workout. They will exercise for a long period of time, watching the calorie counter on the treadmill. But there is a difference between burning 200 calories while walking at a brisk pace and burning 200 calories while performing bursts of high-intensity activity. Because of EPOC, or the after-burn effect, your body will actually burn more calories when you use H.E.A.T. In fact, over a 24-hour period, the total calories burned by one short session of H.E.A.T. is far greater than the total calories burned by an hour of traditional training on a treadmill, stationary bike or stair-climber. And, thanks to EPOC, this means a greater loss of body fat because of the additional calories burned *after* a session of H.E.A.T. Even if more calories are burned during the traditional training in the same scenario, high-energy aerobic training will still win out when it comes to total fat loss after 24 hours.

H.E.A.T. Can Burn Calories for Many Hours After Exercise

Dr. Angelo Tremblay and his colleagues at the Physical Activities Sciences Laboratory at Laval University in Quebec, Canada, challenged the belief that traditional cardiovascular exercise is the best approach for fat loss. Group A did 30 to 45 minutes of moderate-intensity cycling on a stationary bike, four to five times a week for 20 weeks. Group B did sprints on the stationary bike, alternating with short recovery periods, for just 15 weeks. The total amount of time Group B spent exercising varied but was always less than Group A. Group B exercised for shorter sessions over a shorter period of time but experienced *nine times* greater fat loss! They also had significantly elevated levels of HADH, an enzymatic marker of fat burning, showing that they were burning more fat during exercise and at rest afterward. Group A burned more calories while they exercised, but fewer calories after exercising. The opposite was true of Group B. The higher the intensity of the exercise, the greater the energy expenditure after exercise.

Lower Your Triglyceride Levels

In addition to the cholesterol circulating in your blood, you also have circulating fats called serum triglycerides. After you eat, your body converts any extra calories into triglycerides. These are the most common type of fat in the body, and they are a major source of energy. In normal amounts—levels below 150—triglycerides are important to good health. Levels of 200 or above are considered high.

If you regularly eat more calories than you burn, your triglyceride levels may be high. Obese people and those with diabetes are also likely to have high triglycerides. People with high triglycerides tend to have high total cholesterol, elevated levels of LDL ("bad") cholesterol and low levels of HDL ("good") cholesterol. The combination of high triglycerides and low HDL cholesterol is considered a predictor of heart attack. Several clinical studies have shown that people with elevated triglyceride levels have an increased risk of heart disease and stroke.

Fortunately, serum triglycerides can usually be controlled with exercise and changes in diet. Researchers at Southwest Missouri State University and the University of Missouri found that subjects who jogged intermittently on a treadmill after a high-fat meal showed a greater reduction in their serum triglyceride levels than those who jogged continuously. "Our research indicates that regular repetition of short exercise bouts, which add up during a day, have a unique and positive effect on metabolism," said Thomas S. Altena, one of the authors of the study. "People who cannot exercise for long durations due to low fitness levels or busy lifestyles don't have to sit still and wait for a heart attack."

Increase Your Endurance

Another benefit of interval training is that it gets you into better shape than conventional exercise, and it does so more quickly. Many of my clients tell me that switching from conventional exercise to my 4•3•2•1 workouts improved their endurance and stamina dramatically even though they spent less time exercising.

Athletes who are already in great shape are pleased and surprised at their ability to step up their performance after enrolling in the 4•3•2•1 workout program. Adding even occasional bouts of high-intensity interval exercise to a conventional exercise regimen will help you get more out of your cardiovascular workouts. In one recent study, eight women performed seven H.E.A.T. workouts on stationary bicycles over a period of two weeks. When they resumed their regular exercise routine, an hour of continuous moderate cycling, the amount of fat they burned in an hour increased by 36%!

 How H.E.A.T. Can Boost Endurance 100% More than Regular Exercise

At McMaster University in Hamilton, Ontario, Canada, two groups of reasonably fit individuals exercised on stationary bicycles for two weeks and were then evaluated for changes in their endurance levels. Group A consisted of eight participants who performed six sessions of high-intensity cycling. For each session, they alternated between resting and doing 30 seconds of "all-out" sprinting. They sprinted between four and seven times, so the total amount of time they spent exercising was only two to three and a half minutes per session. (This is sometimes called "ultra short" training.) Between sessions, they had a day or two of rest. Group B consisted of another eight subjects who used conventional exercise without sprinting.

After two weeks, the cycle endurance capacity of the subjects in Group A was 100% greater, meaning they had *doubled* their endurance by exercising vigorously for a total of approximately 15 minutes over a period of two weeks. In addition, their resting muscle glycogen content increased by 26%, meaning that in those two weeks their muscles learned to store more energy for use during exercise. The subjects in Group B showed no change in performance. The researchers concluded that short bouts of intense exercise—even as little as 15 minutes over two weeks—produce results comparable to several *weeks* of traditional endurance training.

Benefit from Both Aerobic and Anaerobic Training

When you exercise, your body can use two different metabolic modes to produce the energy you need. The first is *oxidative metabolism,* which your body uses when you perform aerobic exercise such as dancing, jogging or riding a stationary bike. You breathe deeply, taking in plenty of oxygen, and your muscles continue to contract repeatedly without becoming fatigued. The benefits of aerobic exercise include improved circulation, lower blood pressure, greater lung capacity, a stronger heart, increased red blood cells and a reduced risk of cardiovascular disease.

When you perform intense exercise, including sprinting, weight lifting and resistance training, your body can't keep up with the demand for energy if it's using only oxidative metabolism. To keep going, it will shift into *anaerobic metabolism* mode.

Short bursts of intense exercise tax your muscles more and make use of both metabolic modes. With training, your body builds muscle strength and learns to use anaerobic metabolism more effectively, so it can deliver powerful performance on demand.

When you alternate high-intensity exercise with periods of recovery, your body has time to whisk away the lactic acid produced by anaerobic metabolism before a great deal of it can accumulate in your muscles. This preventive measure allows you to put greater demand on your muscles without regretting it the next day.

H.E.A.T. Improves Both Aerobic and Anaerobic Fitness

Members of the Japanese national speed skating team have been using an exercise program involving short, intense workouts for several years. In a study from the National Institute of Fitness and Sports in Japan, seven male physical education majors were asked to ride stationary bikes at moderate intensity for an hour, five days per week for six weeks (traditional cardiovascular exercise). Their aerobic fitness improved somewhat, but their anaerobic fitness did not increase significantly. Next, another seven individuals trained using H.E.A.T., five days per week for six weeks. They alternated between sprinting for 20 seconds at maximum intensity and taking a rest for 10 seconds. At each exercise session, they spent 4 minutes or less actually sprinting. The aerobic fitness of these sprinters improved a remarkable 14%. In addition, they experienced a 28% increase in their anaerobic capacity. Researchers concluded that traditional cardiovascular exercise does not improve anaerobic fitness, but high-intensity interval training improves both aerobic and anaerobic fitness, even in trained athletes.

Boost Your Growth Hormone Levels

Human growth hormone is a naturally secreted hormone that declines over the years, causing the age-related loss of muscle mass called sarcopenia. For this reason, some people jumped to the conclusion that artificially maintaining youthful levels of growth hormone will keep us young—like a fountain of youth but in injection form. Unfortunately, it isn't that simple.

In a 1990 study, a small group of older men received injections of synthetic growth hormone, which caused an increase in their amount of muscle and a decrease in fat. Immediately everyone latched on to the anti-aging properties of growth hormone, even though the authors of the study at no time claimed that it had reversed the aging process. Bodybuilders and others interested in sculpting the appearance of their bodies became particularly intrigued. And, despite the risks, all sorts of people continue to take expensive preparations of synthetic growth hormone, including injections, sprays, creams, "releasers" and "stimulators," because they believe it might build muscle mass, reduce body fat, repair tissues, enhance energy and sexual function, elevate mood and even restore hair color. In other words, they think it will somehow turn back the clock and make them younger. Yet an article in the *New England Journal of Medicine* titled "Can Growth Hormone Prevent Aging?" came to the conclusion that "anti-aging therapy with growth hormone has not been proven effective according to objective outcome criteria."

The fact is, taking synthetic growth hormone can make your muscles bigger but not necessarily stronger, so your body looks impressive but is not actually more fit. Naturally occurring growth hormone, on the other hand, is beneficial for cartilage, bone and muscle growth throughout the body and may protect muscle tissue from being used for energy. H.E.A.T. and resistance training are associated with an elevation in growth hormone levels, which helps to counteract the decreased levels that occur with age. The release of growth hormone increases a few minutes after you begin exercising, then rises sharply when the intensity of the activity increases. All those people who take synthetic growth hormone would be better off exercising.

Women sometimes worry that naturally occurring growth hormone will give them big, bulky unsightly muscles. This is most definitely not the case. Anyone who wants to achieve the prominent muscles of a bodybuilder will have to do a lot more than my 10-minute workouts to get that look.

H.E.A.T. Releases Natural Growth Hormone Even *After* Exercise

A study by researchers at Loughborough University in Leicestershire, England, tested the growth hormone levels of 23 highly trained athletes, both male and female, after they performed an all-out 30-second sprint on a treadmill. The sprint-trained athletes, who trained using H.E.A.T., exhibited three times greater amounts of growth hormone than the endurance-trained athletes, who trained using traditional cardiovascular exercise. Additionally, one hour following exercise, the growth hormone levels in the sprint-trained group were still approximately 10 times higher than their pre-exercise levels. This suggests that H.E.A.T. may increase growth hormone over the long term, which could increase fat metabolism and decrease the metabolism of lean muscle tissue.

Reach Your Peak Performance

In general, skeletal muscles—the muscles that we use for movement—are made up of roughly 50% "slow-twitch" fibers and 50% "fast-twitch" fibers. Each type contracts in a unique way and responds to different kinds of exercise. "Slow-twitch" fibers use oxidative metabolism. They do not tire easily and are used for moderate exercise or prolonged exertion. Marathon runners, for example, usually have more of this type. "Fast-twitch" fibers use both oxidative and anaerobic metabolism. They are better for generating short bursts of strength, but they tire more quickly. Sprinters tend to have more of this type. "Fast-twitch" fibers atrophy with age, which is why older athletes do better at endurance sports.

H.E.A.T. has been used successfully for years to develop peak performance in elite athletes—amateur or professional—but it has not been promoted among the general population until recently. In 2007, an article written by Peter Jaret for *The New York Times* explained that interval exercise was the optimal way to improve performance, noting that it stimulates mitochondria to burn fat before carbohydrates—good news for weight maintenance. In other words, this type of exercise trains your body to become a "fat-burning machine" using fat as the preferred source of fuel for improving energy usage both during longer bouts of exercise and throughout the day.

❸ minutes of Resistance Exercise

The second part of every workout uses compound resistance exercises to tone, firm and tighten your muscles and boost your metabolism. As you already know, alternating periods of vigorous exercise with periods of moderate exercise has a pronounced effect on EPOC. Moreover, resistance training has a greater effect on EPOC than cardiovascular exercise. When you put these two types of exercise together, you get high-intensity resistance training. Like H.E.A.T., compound resistance exercises give you a metabolic boost that continues to burn extra calories even after you finish exercising. This means your metabolism stays elevated for hours, whether or not you stay active. For 3 minutes, you work different muscles of your body using resistance in the form of your own bodyweight, an exercise ball, a medicine ball, flexible bands, dumbbells or barbells.

There are three strengthening exercises in each resistance section: two for the lower body, one for the upper body. You will repeat each exercise for one minute. The number of repetitions you do depends on how strong you are and how difficult the exercise is. It's the size of the weight or the strength of the resistance band you're using that day that counts. Over time, as you get stronger (and you will get stronger, I promise you), you will increase the number of repetitions or increase the difficulty of the exercise. Most likely, both.

After you perform any strengthening exercise, your muscles need time to recover. This is why you do the 10-minute 4•3•2•1 workouts on alternate days. (A safe schedule is built into the daily instructions found in Chapter 10.) Because there are 12 different 4•3•2•1 workouts, you have a wide variety of exercises to choose from. This helps you avoid overtraining any particular muscle (or set of muscles), which in turn helps to prevent soreness after working out. Step-by-step instructions tell you how to perform each routine, but there are three important points to keep in mind when performing any compound resistance exercise:

1. Select a weight (or resistance band) that challenges your muscles but at the same time allows you to perform the movement correctly.

2. Remember to keep your form throughout. Don't sacrifice proper form for speed. Getting sloppy can lead to injury.

3. Don't hold your breath!

The second part of your 4•3•2•1 workout shapes up as follows:

> 60 seconds—as many repetitions as you can do of Exercise 1
> + 60 seconds—as many repetitions as you can do of Exercise 2
> + 60 seconds—as many repetitions as you can do of Exercise 3

= Grand total: ❸ minutes

After completing your 3 minutes of compound resistance exercises, you continue directly to the next part of the workout without resting.

Resistance Exercise Gets You Fit, Fast

When you make compound resistance exercises part of your routine, you don't have to spend long hours in the gym to get beneficial results. An ever-increasing body of research suggests that a short, high-intensity workout can achieve maximum results in less time. Studies show that short sessions of exercise are just as effective, provided you do the exercises correctly and keep up the intensity.

 Resistance Exercise Can Cut Your Gym Time by Two-Thirds

Dr. Julien Baker, a researcher at the Health and Exercise Science Unit at Glamorgan University in Wales, wondered if it was necessary to spend long amounts of time lifting weights. His study involved 16 male weight lifters, who did supervised weight training targeting the upper body three times a week for eight weeks. One group used one set of eight repetitions; the other group used three sets of eight repetitions. Both groups decreased body fat and improved their muscle strength, and no differences were observed between groups. "It's quality over quantity," Dr. Baker included, adding that "it may be better to do a number of regular express workouts, which would fit in with the busy lives that many people lead. . . . To someone starting to exercise, I would recommend they spend less time in the gym, and when they are there, to concentrate on technique."

Resistance Exercise and Weight Loss

If you're interested in weight loss, resistance exercise will help. This section of the 4•3•2•1 workout not only tones your muscles, but also helps you control your weight in three different ways:

1. You burn calories as you exercise.

2. Because of EPOC, you continue to burn calories after you stop exercising.

3. You add muscle tissue to your body, which burns more calories while you're active *and* while you sleep. The more muscle you have, the easier it is to burn excess calories—and the better your body composition will be.

Resistance Exercise Plus Dieting Burns More Fat than Dieting Alone

Dr. Miriam Nelson, director of the prestigious Center for Physical Activity and Nutrition at Tufts

University, notes in her book *Strong Women Stay Slim* that between 25% and 30% of the weight people lose through dieting is actually comprised of water, muscle and other lean tissue, not fat. In addition, she goes on to say that the faster you lose weight, the larger the proportion of nonfat weight loss. For a pilot study, Nelson put 10 overweight women on the same diet, but 5 of them also came into her laboratory twice a week and performed resistance training exercise. By the end of the study, members of both groups had lost about 13 pounds; however, their body composition had changed in different ways. The women in the diet-only group had lost an average of 2.8 pounds of lean tissue. The women who performed strength training had *gained* 1.4 pounds of muscle. This means they really lost 14.6 pounds of fat—or 44% more than the women in the diet-only group. The slight addition of muscle increased their fat-burning capabilities, which went on to boost their metabolism even further!

Resistance Exercise and Aging

For years, most of us thought that weight training was only for professional athletes. Today, it's recommended for healthy individuals of all ages, including many patients with chronic diseases. Resistance training helps to prevent cardiovascular disease and can help prevent as well as manage many other chronic conditions, including lower back pain, osteoporosis, obesity and diabetes.

Resistance exercise is particularly beneficial for older people, especially the frail and elderly. It's never too late to reverse the age-related loss of muscle. Functional exercises help older people with their everyday movements, translating into fewer falls and injuries, which in turn make independence possible. A groundbreaking study by Tufts researcher Dr. Maria Fiatarone showed that patients in nursing homes responded so well to strength training that some of them were able to set aside their canes and walkers!

② minutes of Core-Strengthening Exercises

The third part of the 4•3•2•1 workout involves more strength-training exercises, so technically it's an extension of resistance training and the benefits are the same. However, this part focuses specifically on exercises that strengthen and tone your core, including the muscles of your abdomen, hips and lower back. With these exercises, you will flatten your stomach, strengthen the muscles that surround your trunk and improve your posture.

Some of the core exercises use only bodyweight (sit-ups and crunches, for example), while others are done with inexpensive equipment such as an exercise ball or resistance bands or with free weights or other gym equipment.

Each section of core exercises includes two exercise routines. You perform as many repetitions of each exercise as you can, without losing the correct form, for 60 seconds.

Core-Strengthening Exercises Can Reduce Lower Back Pain

Forty-four people who were suffering from chronic lower back pain were randomly assigned to two treatment groups in a study conducted at the Curtin University of Technology in Perth, Australia. The individuals assigned to Group A performed core-strengthening exercises and after 10 weeks showed a significant reduction in the intensity of their back pain as well as in their functional disability levels. These improvements were still apparent at a 30-month follow-up. On the other hand, the individuals in Group B underwent other commonly prescribed conservative treatments that were directed by their medical practitioner. These participants demonstrated no significant change in back pain or functional disability after intervention or at follow-up.

The core-strengthening section of your 4•3•2•1 workout will go like this:

60 seconds—as many repetitions as you can do of Exercise 1 (for stomach)

+ 60 seconds—as many repetitions as you can do of Exercise 2 (for back and/or hips)

= Grand total: ❷ minutes

After completing your 2 minutes of core-strengthening exercises, you continue directly to the next part of the workout without resting.

Here's something to keep in mind: The stronger your core, the stronger you will be in everything you do, from just getting out of a chair or walking to the store to competing in sports or dancing the tango. As an added benefit, strengthening the muscles of your abdomen, hips and lower back helps to prevent back problems. Four out of five adults will have back pain at some point in their lives. I'd like you to be in the 20% of people who do not have this problem. Besides, a stronger core means you'll stand taller, walk with more spring in your step and look better in your clothes.

❶ minute of Stretching and Deep Breathing

The 4•3•2•1 workout wraps up with 1 minute of stretching exercises and deep breathing— the perfect way to oxygenate your brain and nourish your muscles. These stretching and breathing exercises are the perfect antidote to stress and fatigue. They help you feel renewed and rejuvenated in mind and body before resuming your day. You may enjoy them so much that you'll use them at other times, too.

Stretching After Exercise Speeds Recovery

The concept of stretching may seem simple, but there's more to the subject than you might expect. Several studies showed that static stretching immediately before exercising actually reduces performance in certain activities and also can lead to muscle injury, especially when you overstretch (or stretch until it hurts). The best way to prepare for vigorous exercise is to do a gentle warm-up activity like walking at an easy pace.

The latest research shows that stretching should be performed *after* warming up or *after* working out. Following a workout, stretching helps to prevent soreness by reducing the amount of lactic acid that builds up in your muscles with exertion, so you feel

less stiff the next day. Along with deep breathing, it allows you to recover from exercising and leaves you physically and mentally rested for the next set or workout.

Stretching After Exercising Improves Performance

Dr. Ian Shrier, an expert in sports medicine, performed a meta-analysis of 23 articles related to stretching and performance. The research shows that stretching immediately before exercise does not improve force or jump height. On the other hand, stretching on a regular basis—not immediately before exercise—improves force, jump height, and speed. Dr. Shrier concluded, "If one stretches, one should stretch after exercise or at a time not related to exercise."

Stretching Is a Form of Exercise in Its Own Right

Done on a regular basis, stretching has a number of benefits for your heath. It relieves stress, helps to alleviate aches and pains, and keeps you limber, making it easier to perform daily activites such as picking up the newspaper or reaching to replace a lightbulb. It improves your posture, balance and coordination, and prevents injury by loosening muscles that are stiff or tight. And it enhances circulation, oxygenating your cells and assisting with all body processes.

When you perform a 4•3•2•1 workout every other day or so, you get the short-term benefits of post-exercise stretching, as well as the long-term benefits of stretching on a regular basis.

Deep Breathing Increases Oxygen Intake and Lowers Blood Pressure

Each time you perform a 10-minute workout, you practice deep breathing and reap its rewards. Taking deep breaths fills your lungs and allows a more complete exchange of old and new air. A "cleansing breath" is a deep breath of air that you take in slowly through your nose and exhale slowly through your mouth.

When asked to breathe deeply, some people will raise their shoulders, puff out their chest and inhale sharply. Taking a big chest breath is not the same as deep abdominal breathing, which makes your belly rise and fall. If you've never tried this type of breathing before, place a hand on your belly and imagine that you're pushing it away from you as you inhale deeply. (Remember to start by exhaling—you can't fill up your lungs unless you exhale first!)

Deep breathing enhances the oxygen supply to your cells, helping them burn more fat and giving you more energy. It also helps to keep fluids running through the lymph system, which is an essential part of getting rid of toxins and cellular debris. In addition, it can help bring down blood pressure levels. When someone has high blood pressure, even a small, sustained drop can make a difference when it comes to improving the condition. Some people with

high blood pressure would rather not take medication to correct it. Other people, despite medication, have not been successful at meeting their blood pressure goal. In these cases, deep breathing can provide substantial health benefits.

Deep Breathing Helps to Control Blood Pressure

In a study at Chicago's Rush University, 89 people with high blood pressure received a computerized musical device to help them learn how to lower their breathing rate. The patients who used it the most—about 15 minutes per day for eight weeks—had a 15-point drop in blood pressure!

Deep Breathing Calms You Down

Scientific studies have demonstrated that deep breathing triggers the relaxation response and calms the nervous system. In the short term, breathing deeply can help you focus your attention, keep you from losing your temper and make it easier to fall asleep. Over the long term, practicing deep breathing on a regular basis helps you stay healthy by reducing stress and anxiety.

The medical community sometimes refers to slow, controlled breathing as *paced respiration.* Because deep breathing can release endorphins, those neurotransmitters that act like a natural painkiller, patients are encouraged to use paced respiration to ease their anxiety associated with dental work or medical examinations. Cardiac patients are asked to use paced respiration to slow down their heart rate, and women approaching menopause are advised to use it to help with hot flashes. It also helps motion sickness.

Gaining and Losing: Why Diets Don't Work

At the beginning of this chapter, you met twin sisters Jill and Laura, who were anxious to lose some weight in time for a class reunion. As you'll remember, while Jill resumed dieting and working out on the treadmill, Laura made an appointment with me to find out more about the 10-Minute Total Body Breakthrough. Because I have had so much experience with clients in Laura's situation, I wanted to save her from her sister's fate. She had the motivation to succeed, but she still had a lot to learn about the principles of gaining and losing weight.

The Life and Death of Fat Cells

When you think of a fat cell, picture a tiny plastic balloon holding a droplet of butter. Believe it or not, you have more than 40 billion fat cells in your body; if you're obese, you have two or three times that number. These billions of balloon-like fat cells are responsible for two primary functions: storing energy and providing energy. When you take in more calories than you use, your fat cells store the extra energy for later. When you take in fewer calories than you need, your fat cells release stored fatty acids into your bloodstream. Even when no food is available, your bodily processes can continue without interruption until you're able to eat again.

Fat cells can expand or shrink, depending on whether food is abundant or in short supply. Altogether, your fat cells are capable of storing hundreds of pounds of energy. When food is plentiful, the cells expand. If an individual keeps overeating, they grow and grow until they look as if they're about to pop. When they reach their limit, they don't divide the way other body cells do; instead, they send out a signal to nearby immature cells to start producing more fat cells.

Fat cells are also extremely long-lived. You might even have heard that fat cells never die. A 2008 article in *The New York Times* by Gina Kolata tried to get to the bottom of this myth, explaining that every year 10% of your fat cells do, in fact, die; however, they're replaced by new fat cells, which means the total number of fat cells in your body remains the same. In general, if you lose weight, your fat cells shrink, but they don't disappear. Liposuction reduces the number of these cells, but weight gain can still occur in other areas as the remaining fat cells expand.

The life and death of fat cells is a very complicated subject, but the important concept here is that fat cells, under certain circumstances, will give up their energy and shrink.

Whatever your weight might be, you can adapt the 10-Minute Total Body Breakthrough program to your specific needs:

- If you think you're too skinny, you can put on muscle mass.

- If you're the right weight but have the wrong percentage of body fat, you can shrink your fat cells and restore muscle, transforming your health and appearance without changing the numbers on the scale.

- If, over time, you have accumulated some extra weight, you can use the principles of "traffic light" eating and the 10-minute workouts sensibly and gradually to lose the extra fat until you reach your goal.

Putting Your Metabolism to Work for You

Most people think of metabolism in terms of burning calories—in particular, how many calories they use on a daily basis. Some people seem to be blessed with a "good" metabolism that allows them to drink milk shakes and eat chocolate cream pie. But metabolism is not a fixed number. If you're not one of those lucky people who can eat whatever they want, take heart. There is a great deal you can do to make your metabolism work for you.

Your metabolism is, among other things, a balancing act between constructive and destructive activities. All of the thousands of biochemical processes that are simultaneously occurring in your body can be lumped together under two main headings: anabolism (building up) and catabolism (breaking down). Molecules are built up so energy is stored; food is broken down so energy is released. Cells, tissues and proteins are built up; nutrients are broken down.

Three separate processes determine the number of calories your body needs each day:

1. **Your resting metabolic rate, or RMR.** This represents the number of calories that your body needs for basic functions such as breathing and is influenced by how much muscle you have. Men tend to have more lean body mass (muscle) than women, so in general they will burn more calories, even during sleep. Sarcopenia, or age-related loss of muscle mass, causes a decline in RMR—*unless* strength training is used to keep muscles strong. RMR accounts for approximately 70% of the total number of calories your body burns in a day.

2. **The thermic effect of food, or TEF (also called thermogenesis).** This is a fancy way of describing the number of calories your body uses to digest, absorb and metabolize the food you eat. TEF accounts for approximately 10% of the total number of calories your body burns in a day. It's the reason celery is technically a negative-calorie food—you burn more calories chewing, digesting and absorbing the nutrients in the food than are found in the food itself. Ice water also uses up more calories than it provides, because your body derives no calories from water but must expend energy to warm it up. Unfortunately, this does not work as a weight-loss tip, because the number of calories required is minimal.

3. **Your level of physical activity and exercise.** Moving your muscles requires energy. The more you move, the more calories you burn. Physical activity accounts for approximately 20% of the total number of calories your body burns in a day—but this number can vary a great deal between individuals. This is why exercise is so important!

If you take in more calories than you use up during the day—that is, if you eat too much—you put on fat. Too much fat is unhealthy, but a little bit provides your body with an emergency supply of energy. In women, fat cells create the hormone estrogen. Women whose estrogen levels are about to plummet as they approach menopause sometimes develop a "menopot" (a small amount of belly fat),

Exercise More, Eat More

When you read the labels on packaged foods, the "percent daily value" figures are based on an average diet of 2,000 calories per day. Whether you would gain or lose weight on 2,000 calories a day depends on how many calories your body actually needs. This is where exercise comes in. If you eat more than your body needs, you can burn up the extra calories with exercise before they have a chance to turn into fat. Athletes can consume 6,000 calories a day without getting fat, partly because of their active lifestyle and partly because they have more muscle, which uses up more energy. Olympic gold medalist Michael Phelps consumed 12,000 calories a day in training—without including any chocolate or wine. But he also swam up to 50 miles a week!

which is nature's way of ensuring that the body still has some estrogen. Too much fat, however, may result in enough extra estrogen to cause hormone-related problems.

If you're carrying extra fat, you can burn it off with exercise—but only if you take in fewer calories than your body needs so that it's forced to dip into its energy reserves. Unfortunately for all the dieters out there, it takes a *lot* of exercise to burn off all the calories in a sugar cookie. If you're looking at the calorie counter on your treadmill, you could easily get discouraged. (I could insert a table here that shows exactly how many minutes you would have to exercise to burn off a specific number of calories, but this book is about focusing on fitness for the rest of your life without an unhealthy preoccupation with calorie counts.)

Some athletes get in the habit of living large while they're young and active—especially football players, who are encouraged to be big. When these athletes get older and their level of activity declines, they may continue to consume the same number of calories. We've all seen what happens next. All those calories that are no longer getting burned are stored as fat. I'm thinking of a phys ed teacher I had when I was a kid. He was a standout athlete in his youth, but he had lost his muscles and put on pounds of fat by the time he came to our school. He could still throw a football, but in class he just stood in the middle of the gym and blew his whistle while we did all the exercise.

While it's true that extra calories will make you fat, it does not automatically follow that eating fewer calories will make you thin. Strange, isn't it? This is where it pays to know a little more about how to manipulate your metabolism.

Why Dieting Alone Will Never Work

Your body constantly strives for balance and harmony. When confronted by any threat, whether it's a virus, extreme temperature or an injury, your body pays a huge price just to get back to its comfort zone.

Unhealthy dieting has the same costly effect. When you severely restrict the number of calories you take in, your cells get the message that you're starving. This challenge to your body is not taken lightly. A warning light flashes and biochemical changes begin to take place within your fat cells and throughout the rest of your body.

Here's what happens when you diet:

- **Your metabolism slows down.** Your body sees the lack of nutrients as a threat and begins to conserve energy by decreasing your metabolism by as much as 40%.

- **Your body activates special fat-storing enzymes.** Your body is trying to store more fat to ensure your survival. Researchers have measured the production of the fat-storing enzymes and found that their number doubles during a very low-calorie diet. This means your body is now working twice as hard to store fat and is able to store twice as much fat as it did before you went on a diet!

- **Your body reduces its fat-burning enzymes.** Research has also shown that when you go on a very low-calorie diet, levels of fat-burning enzymes are lowered by as much as 50%. This makes you even more susceptible to gaining fat, both during and after the diet. This is a huge problem when you want to lose weight all over again in the future.

- **You lose muscle tissue.** Extreme dieting is the fastest way to lose muscle. When you restrict your calorie intake, your body begins to search for any readily available source of energy. It draws energy from your muscles, making them smaller, weaker and less efficient at burning fat, both during and after your diet. Low levels of glucose cause your body to burn the protein in your muscles for energy. This means that as you lose weight, you are really losing a combination of fat, water and muscle. With less metabolically active muscle tissue, it's harder for you to burn calories.

The Keys Study: The Psychological Price of Extreme Dieting

In this 1950 study, Ancel Keys and his research group began by recruiting 36 young men who were fit and psychologically sound. For the first three months, the participants ate normally. For the next six months, their calories were cut in half (just like many weight-loss diets today). During this period, they became preoccupied with food, developed weird food rituals and started hoarding odd objects. They also developed emotional problems, such as mood swings and depression, and their interest in sex waned. They lost, on average, approximately 25% of their former weight. Their resting metabolic rate dropped 40%.

The final three months of the yearlong study were devoted to rehabilitation. The young men could eat freely again, but their eating patterns and psychological health did not immediately return to normal. Constantly hungry, they would lose control of their eating and then feel guilty. Many of them engaged in bingeing and purging. Emotionally, they still experienced upheaval, and it took eight months for all of the men to regain their interest in sex.

The Semi-Starvation Study, published in 1950 by Ancel Keys and his colleagues at the University of Minnesota, was the first to show that extreme dieting also has devastating effects on our mental health. This study remains the gold standard among research projects concerning psychological changes that result from restricting calories, but newer studies echo its findings. A 1993 article from the *Annals of Internal Medicine,* entitled "Relation of Dieting and Voluntary Weight Loss to Psychological Functioning and Binge Eating," notes that "more conventional, self-initiated dieting is also associated with adverse psychological effects in young women of normal weight." Although obese patients feel less depressed when they go on a diet, "dieting by persons of normal weight is associated with low self-esteem and depressive symptoms" and "is linked to the development and maintenance of eating disorders such as anorexia nervosa and bulimia nervosa."

The bottom line is that restricting calories alone is *not* the way to get fit. The 10-Minute Total Body Breakthrough program will enable you to lose fat without losing muscle or experiencing any of the other hazards of dieting.

Being Thin Is Not the Same as Being Fit

To develop the best body you've ever had, you need to exercise—and the great news is that you don't have to spend hours on the treadmill. Let's take a last look at Jill and Laura, the twin sisters who took entirely different approaches to losing weight and getting in shape for their upcoming class reunion. Over a three-month period, they each worked hard on their fitness regimens but with very different results.

Four days a week, Jill walked on the treadmill at the gym for up to an hour, and she signed up for machine training at the gym once a week for 45 minutes. Her goal was to use the treadmill for an hour each day, but she found it monotonous and boring and often did not do the full 60 minutes. She also went back on the South Beach diet. Jill found herself constantly thinking about food and feeling guilty about eating the wrong things. After three months of this routine, she was feeling unmotivated—maybe trying to look as good as Debbie Meyers wasn't *really* worth the effort. She couldn't wait for the whole ordeal to be over.

Laura trained the 4•3•2•1 way. Every day, she spent at least 10 minutes doing something active. On Mondays, Wednesdays and Fridays, she did a 4•3•2•1 workout. On the other days, she chose 10 minutes of different physical activities. She did not diet, but she ate the right foods and increased her consumption of fruits and vegetables. Three months later, Laura was lean, fit and healthy. She could wear clothes she hadn't worn in years and could fit into her daughter's jeans. Laura was getting lots of compliments from friends and family, which she enjoyed, but what she really liked was the way she felt. She has no intention of stopping her 10-minute workouts!

Comparing Jill's and Laura's Experiences with
Conventional and 4·3·2·1 Fitness Programs

After 12 Weeks	Jill's Results Conventional Approach	Laura's Results 4·3·2·1 Approach
Hours each week spent exercising	At least 4 hours a week at the gym	70 minutes per week at home or outdoors
Changes in fitness level	Feels the same.	Lost 2.5 inches off her waist. Lost 4.2 inches off her hips. Decreased body fat by 6%. Improved endurance. Increased strength.
Weight loss	5 pounds	14 pounds (actually more, if you allow for her gain of new muscle tissue)
Energy level	Feels tired most of the time.	Feels fantastic.
Personal status	Can't wear her "skinny" clothes. Struggling with confidence. Thinking about skipping the reunion.	Wears smaller sizes. Feels as good as she did 20 years ago. Looking forward to the reunion and whatever else life brings.
Nutritional status	Starving, cranky Feels deprived.	Not hungry Enjoys her favorite foods.

chapter 5

A New Look at Nutrition

Food as High-Octane Fuel

Have you ever gone to someone's house for a special dinner and wondered: What *is* this stuff? I once attended a Thanksgiving feast in New Orleans that included turducken (a chicken inside a duck inside a turkey), oyster stuffing, eggplant-and-shrimp casserole and sweet potato pie. The food couldn't have tasted better, but it didn't feel like Thanksgiving without my mom's cranberry mold.

We all love foods that we grew up with—we're used to their tastes and they bring us comfort. But we also go along eating the same dishes, prepared according to the same recipes, because repeating what's familiar is always easier than change. It takes some determination to change our eating habits. And it takes commitment. But very soon you'll develop a taste for healthy food—and once the compliments start coming in you'll find it easier to turn down a bowl of mac 'n cheese in favor of a salad.

Food as Fuel: It's About Energy

Food is energy. We *like* food because it tastes good, but we *need* food for energy. That's why I encourage you to think of food as fuel—a way to keep your engine running smoothly all day.

We've all had the experience of sitting in our car, stuck in traffic, and suddenly noticing that the fuel gauge on the dashboard is pointing toward Empty. As soon as possible, we head for the nearest gas station, hoping and praying the car doesn't go silent and roll to a stop by the edge of the road. And if we get there in time, we fill up the gas tank with the car's only source of energy: gasoline. (For the purpose of this example, let's leave experimental and hybrid vehicles aside.) We wouldn't put window cleaner or dish detergent in the tank and expect the car to run properly. Would you fill your tank with 10 gallons of diet soda or chocolate syrup and expect it to take you to your mother-in-law's house 100 miles away?

Just like a car, your body needs the *right* fuel to run smoothly, and this means the best combination of protein, carbohydrates and fats. These nutrients allow you to move, think, feel and perform your best.

When you think of food as fuel, the best choices become very clear. Whenever you're about to put food in your mouth, you'll ask yourself: Am I eating this *for energy* or *for enjoyment*? For example, if you finish a scrumptious dinner and then want to eat popcorn at the movies, you're dealing with a desire to eat food for enjoyment, not for energy. If you argue with a friend and then have the urge to eat ice cream, you're dealing with emotional eating, not eating for energy. (For more about emotional eating, see page 53.) If you're having trouble concentrating and are feeling tired, lightheaded and/or irritable, you could eat for enjoyment (say, a fat-filled snack with a sugar-loaded drink that will cause you to crash in a couple of hours) or you could eat for energy (a piece of fruit or a healthy snack with some lean protein that will keep you going).

Why This Plan Works for Everyone

It doesn't matter if you're already following a specific nutritional program; all the ideas in this chapter will work for you, too. Truly, whether you're eating according to a doctor-prescribed, sports-specific or popular weight management plan, thinking of food as fuel will help you achieve your goals.

When you learn how to use food as fuel, you will eat in a way that helps you stay mentally, physically and emotionally in balance all day. Your energy level and your ability to concentrate will not go through peaks and crashes like the stock market. You'll also lose extra fat, overcome emotional eating and help your body's metabolism begin working for you instead of against you.

Even though eating unfamiliar foods can be a big adjustment, my clients on the 10-Minute Total Body Breakthrough program quickly feel so much better, and have so much more energy, that they find it easy to stick with their new eating habits. Conventional wisdom holds that lasting change takes 21 days of training, so it might take a couple of weeks for you to feel comfortable with your new food choices, but I promise you'll feel so much better that you'll never go back to your old way of eating.

My goal is to help you become fit, energetic and strong. This means not only encouraging you to *get moving* every day, but also helping you learn how to eat in a healthy way for life—not just for the next six months or until you reach your target weight, but for however many years you've got left.

The rest of this chapter will explain the three fueling strategies that I came up with in developing a fun, simple approach to healthy eating. They're easy to remember:

1. Be Real

2. Eat Real

3. Get Real

1. Be Real

Your goal is not to eat in a prescribed manner for a short period of time—that is, to "diet"—but to establish new eating habits for life. Healthy eating has far-reaching effects, including weight loss and abundant energy. Good nutrition boosts your immune system, keeps your bones strong and stabilizes your moods. People who make poor choices about food tend to look drawn and fatigued, with dark circles under their eyes and grayish skin. Conversely, you can tell people who eat healthy foods by their bright eyes, clear skin, gleaming teeth, strong fingernails and thick, shining hair.

The basic principles of using food as fuel stay the same whether you want to lose, gain or maintain weight. If you need to put on a few pounds, you use the same approach but eat more; if your goal is weight loss, you just eat less. I like this approach for many reasons, including the fact that it eliminates all the negatives of the dieting mentality. If weight loss is your goal, combining the 4•3•2•1 program with the fueling strategies in this chapter will help you lose weight painlessly, without feeling hungry, deprived or irritable.

Like any father, I am concerned about the messages the media are sending to my kids, especially my daughter. Will she grow up thinking that she's not worthy of love and admiration unless she wears a size zero? That people who are heavy lack willpower and deserve to be treated with contempt? That it's better to be skinny than to be fit and healthy?

This is no way to look at life. I have seen grown women (and some men) literally starving themselves, skipping meals, vomiting after meals, popping diet pills, even taking up smoking, in order to lose weight. When the number on the bathroom scale rises, their inner critic says: "You really blew it! You're no good! Now you can't eat for a week!" If you're hearing a voice like that, it's time to ditch the scale and *be real* about eating.

Here's an idea: Instead of looking at the scale, review your day every evening and take note of all the things you did right. Focus on the activities and food choices that benefited you the most. Plan healthier activities and food decisions for tomorrow. Build on your successes, and a new, slimmer, stronger, happier and more energetic *you* will appear before you know it.

The Diet Mentality

Dieting usually involves looking for a quick fix to a problem that took time to develop. Unhealthy diets don't allow you to *be real* about food, and they're full of danger. Besides destroying muscle tissue, lowering metabolism, increasing fat-storing enzymes and causing harmful "yo-yo" weight loss inevitably followed by weight gain, dieting has a number of negative effects on your mindset.

- Dieting makes you hungry and keeps you preoccupied with food all day long.
- Dieting forces you to focus on your weight—a number on a scale—rather than on your health and fitness.

- Diets perpetuate a negative self-image.
- Dieting creates an unnatural relationship with eating and makes all food seem like an ever-present enemy that keeps you constantly on your guard.

- Dieting takes control of your food choices away from you. By identifying forbidden foods, dieting causes feelings of deprivation.
- Dieting causes self-defeating feelings of guilt and shame when you eat the "wrong" foods.

The Pros and Cons of Counting Calories

You probably know people who can tell you the precise calorie count of hundreds of different foods. But knowing the number of calories in a kumquat is not the kind of knowledge you need to be healthy. Calories tell you nothing about a food's nutritional value or how your body will use it.

I'm not saying calories don't count; they do. For example, you should know that a 12-ounce can of regular soda has 150 completely useless calories. For the same number of calories, you could eat *real* food with *real* nutrients: two cups of fresh pineapple containing 160 mg of vitamin C; or one large banana with 420 mg of potassium; or five large carrots with 60,140 IUs of vitamin A.

In addition, calorie counts can be misleading. It's possible for a food with *fewer* calories to make

How to Get Fuel *and* Enjoyment from 150 Calories

There's a lot more to fueling your body than counting calories. Dieters who obsess over calorie counts but ignore good nutrition are sabotaging their health and fitness. Instead of reaching for a soda or mocha latte, try a snack that contains 150 calories but provides you with both nutrients and enjoyment:

3 large peaches	1 strawberry yogurt
5 strawberries dipped in dark chocolate	1 6" corn tortilla with 2 tablespoons of bean dip and a splash of salsa
1 medium apple with 1 tablespoon peanut butter	1 6" whole-wheat pita pocket with 2 ounces water-packed tuna and 1 tablespoon light dressing
½ cup shelled edamame (soybeans)	
2 slices of whole-wheat bread	½ cup cooked pasta with ½ cup vegetables, 1 tablespoon feta cheese and 2 tablespoons light dressing
1 whole-wheat English muffin	
½ chicken breast	

you gain weight! Two slices of diet white bread have fewer calories than two slices of whole-grain bread. But the diet bread, made with white flour, is quickly converted by your body into sugar, which can force your system into fat-storing mode. The whole-grain bread, on the other hand, is digested more slowly, giving you energy over a long period of time.

When you learn how to *be real* about food, you steadily give your body the fuel it needs without alternately bingeing and starving. You make sensible choices throughout the day so you never end up ravenously hungry at the grocery store, wondering what's for dinner and what you can eat in the car before you even get home. You learn how to tell when your body is hungry and you need to "fuel up."

By using the concept of the 0–10 fuel gauge on the opposite page throughout the day, you can train yourself to be aware of your need for energy and to fuel your body accordingly. This seems like a simple idea, but most people do not fuel themselves appropriately. Many skip breakfast and even lunch, letting themselves get so hungry that later they eat more than they need. Some dieters will ignore their hunger until they faint, or get so hungry that they make poor food choices. Other people eat at the first sign of hunger or even *before* they feel hungry. Many routinely eat past the point of just feeling comfortable.

As a child, you depended on others to feed you. You may never have had enough food, or you may have had too much. You may remember being told to clean your plate and to think of all the starving children in Africa, or China, or whatever country your family chose. When, what and how much you ate was not really up to you. It's time to retrain yourself to fuel your body appropriately and to stop when you're comfortable (level 5 on the fuel gauge).

Moderation, Not Deprivation

You intuitively know that sweet desserts have lots of calories and don't do much for you nutritionally—that these foods are for enjoyment, not for energy. But this does not mean you have to deprive yourself. As long as you're using food as fuel (replenishing your

Your Fuel Gauge: Eating for Energy

Think of your stomach as a gas tank with a handy fuel gauge. What would it read right now? How important is it for you to eat at this moment?

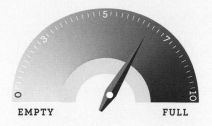

EMPTY   FULL

0   Empty stomach, nagging headache; need fuel urgently!

3   Stomach growling, hunger pangs; need to fuel.

5   Comfortable; fueled and physically satisfied.

7   Uncomfortably full; did not need to eat so much.

10   Stuffed—loosen the belt, it's Thanksgiving all over again!

body's need for energy), it is completely appropriate to have a treat once in a while. If you're attending a family dinner and Grandma Eloise has made her famous chocolate velvet fudge cake, it's okay to honor her cooking by having a piece. However, since the goal is to *be real*, you may want to avoid sugar the following day and bring your eating back into balance.

Food should be experienced and enjoyed. Life is all about fluctuation and change, so taking a rigid approach to food is like using a ruler to measure an apple or swimming straight through a lake instead of enjoying the walk around it. When you're realistic about food, you can flex your eating to accommodate real life. If someone takes you out to dinner at a five-star restaurant, are you going to say "no" to the taste experiences of a lifetime? I hope not. If someone brings your favorite birthday cake, are you going to eat the whole thing today, then starve yourself tomorrow? Please don't!

Many people have told me the same secret: that sometimes they eat a pint of ice cream for dinner and nothing else. I understand the rationale. If you eat a "bad" food and nothing else, the calories will come out the same and no harm is done. But watch out—this is a trap! To your body, 200 calories of ice cream is *not* the same as 200 calories of nutritious fruits, vegetables, whole grains and protein. Limiting your healthy foods never makes up for eating a large amount of an indulgence food.

Believe it or not, most Americans are overfed but undernourished. We don't receive the necessary nutrients, and we're left scouring the pantry for that special something. Satisfy your body's genuine need for energy before eating for enjoyment. If you have the urge for ice cream, eat a nutritious dinner—then have your treat. You'll have the best of both worlds.

Top 10 Signs of the Diet Mentality

1. "How many calories are in that seafood platter?"
2. "This looks good, but I can't have any."
3. "Today I get to eat anything I want!"
4. "I won't have anything except water until it's time for dinner."
5. "I have clothes in my closet ranging all the way from size 10 to size 20."
6. "After the reunion, I'm having an ice cream sundae with everything on it!"
7. "Hey, I hit my target weight! Now I can stop exercising!"
8. "I haven't lost any weight in a week. Tomorrow I'll do an extra two hours of cardio."
9. "I just weighed myself, and I feel worthless."
10. "I am so *hungry*."

The Ups and Downs of Emotional Eating

Emotional eating can ruin your attempts to maintain your ideal weight or to lose weight—and the worst part is, you might not even realize it's happening. When I ask my clients what they've had to eat, they'll tell me about their meals and snacks but won't mention the bag of chips in the car, or the candy jar

Stress-Related Eating Problems

Three things can happen when you're feeling stressed:

1. *You lose interest in eating.* And then, when you can finally relax, your appetite comes back and you're so hungry that you can't help making regrettable food choices.

2. *You focus on eating as a way to avoid thinking about your problems.* You may even use eating to procrastinate. (If you have to start doing your income taxes, you might find that you need a muffin first!)

3. *You use food to relax.* A full stomach is calming. Also, when you eat carbohydrates, your insulin levels rise in order to manage the increase in blood sugar. This process raises our levels of tryptophan, the amino acid precursor of serotonin, with the result that production of serotonin increases in the brain. Many of us get a craving for sweets when we're stressed or anxious, which may be our body's subconscious attempt to raise our serotonin levels. A big dose of comforting carbohydrates, whether it's a bowl of ice cream or a bowl of mashed potatoes, really does make you feel better—but remember portion control!

at work, or the bucket of popcorn at the scary movie. These people aren't trying to be deceitful. It's just that most of the time this kind of emotional eating is off the radar.

Everyone engages in emotional eating, but some people have less control over this issue than others. Below are some helpful suggestions for overcoming emotional overeating.

■ **Get a handle on your stress.** Stress can lead to emotional eating, which in turn can lead to feeling guilty or out of control—more stress! Practice the stress management techniques in the daily instructions beginning on page 236. Consider repeating the stretching and deep breathing section at the end of each 10-minute workout. Being active every day will help. So will sharing your highs and lows with trusted friends or family members. Instead of eating high-calorie comfort foods, see if you can figure out what's eating you. Use your journal, or a small tape recorder, to note your feelings throughout the day.

■ **Remember your fuel gauge.** Before eating anything, ask yourself: "What do I really need?" If it's for energy, by all means eat. But if your body doesn't really need fuel, then what is it that you're searching for? Take a moment to experience your emotions and identify what you truly need.

■ **Be intentional about eating.** Appreciating what you eat makes a difference. Don't eat while you're busy doing something else, whether it's working, driving or watching TV. Unconscious eating can sabotage all your efforts to get fit.

■ **Keep a food diary for three days.** Write down everything you eat, and record your fuel gauge level (from 0 to 10) before and after eating, as well as any emotions you may be feeling. Identify any self-defeating thoughts, and those times when your inner critic is loudest. Often when you see your emotions and eating habits written down in black and white, connections become clear.

■ **Prepare "emergency" snacks ahead of time.** Keep healthy snacks that you enjoy on hand, in case you get the urge to splurge. Portion them out into little plastic bags for guilt-free snacking. When the bag is empty, you stop.

■ **Nurture yourself with enjoyment other than food.** If you're out of no-calorie ideas, see the list on page 52.

■ **Join a support group.** Professional coaching can help you work through your emotional eating patterns. Go to www.4321fitness.com or www.oa.org.

2. Eat Real

Recently I saw a product on the shelf that really made me shake my head. It was a "fruit spread" with an enticing picture of fruit on the front, and it was advertised as calorie-free, carb-free, fat-free and sugar-free. I was curious how this product could have virtually nothing useful for your body, so I looked at the label. The number one ingredient was water (okay, technically that's useful), followed by artificial flavors, a sugar substitute, cellulose gel, xanthan thickener, coloring and preservatives. It was being advertised as "perfect for the health-conscious and health-concerned consumer."

Excuse me?

What you want to do is give your body *real* food to work with: complex carbohydrates to burn for energy, healthy fats to form cell membranes, quality protein to build tissues, and so on. You want to eat more healthy nutrients, less sugar and fewer chemical additives. Small changes add up, and over time they have a huge impact on your energy level as well as your waist size.

I once asked a highly respected dietitian and health professional, "If you could share only one piece of advice with your clients to help them improve their health through nutrition, what would it be?" Without hesitation, she said, "*Eat real*—real food!" She pointed out that we settle for imitation, processed, boxed, packaged products devoid of nutrients and loaded with chemicals and empty calories. These "fake" foods have been stripped of their nutrients and reconstructed for convenience to last for months on store shelves.

When you *eat real*, you consume the original whole food in as close to its natural state as possible. My first choice is always nutrient-rich natural foods, those that can be raised, picked, gathered, milked or caught without significant processing or packaging. Choose nutrient-dense foods that have health benefits in every calorie, instead of

Eat Small, Eat Often

Schedule appointments with yourself to fuel your body five or six times a day: three meals and two or three snacks at regular intervals (breakfast, snack, lunch, snack, dinner . . . late snack optional). Research supports eating small, frequent meals throughout the day to keep your blood sugar levels stable. Even if this is the only change you make, it would be a great improvement over eating a few large meals, which causes fluctuations in your blood sugar and forces your body to alternate between fat burning and fat storing. When you're careful to eat foods that are digested slowly and used for fuel over several hours, you avoid sugar highs and lows, keep your metabolic rate high, and improve your energy level and alertness. Some studies have even reported that people who consume frequent small meals and snacks (every three hours) have less body fat than individuals who eat a few large meals.

Many, many people tell me that they skip breakfast because their stomach just isn't "awake" in the morning. This is because during the night, as you sleep, your body digests any remaining food from the day before, then switches over to fat-burning mode. Now that you're up and beginning your busy day, you need fuel. If you think you're doing just fine without breakfast, I challenge you to make yourself eat breakfast every day for a week and then reassess how you feel about it. I guarantee you will find that eating small meals and snacks throughout the day, including breakfast, gives you more energy with less hunger and fewer cranky periods.

If you're really organized, you can plan your meals and snacks for the entire week. Anticipate tricky situations that might throw you off schedule, then plan how to handle them so you don't go for extended periods without food. If you don't plan for success, you plan to fail.

foods that have lots of calories but few nutrients. Pick foods with quality protein, wholesome carbohydrates, healthy fats, and plenty of vitamins, minerals, enzymes, antioxidants and phytochemicals to refresh, rejuvenate and renew your cells, enhance your immune system, prevent disease, improve your mood, increase your energy, keep your mind sharp and promote all-around vibrant health.

Real Food

To get started, stick with foods that you really like!—the foods that bring you the most satisfaction and enjoyment. But be sure to select healthy versions of those items. Choose foods that are:

- *Unrefined, unprocessed* and *unbleached.* The more processed a food is, the fewer nutrients it has left.

- *Fresh,* and preferably grown locally. Micronutrients are lost when foods travel long distances or are held in storage for long periods of time.

- *High-fiber.* Fiber takes the edge off hunger, provides bulk for the gastrointestinal tract, works to keep blood sugar levels stable and helps prevent heart disease and other illnesses.

- *Lean, reduced-fat, low-fat or nonfat.* You can easily reduce the amount of saturated fat in your diet by buying lean cuts of meat, choosing skinless chicken and switching to low-fat dairy products. (For more about "good" and "bad" fats, see the opposite page.)

- *Low GI (glycemic index),* meaning they do not cause a rapid rise in blood sugar.

- *Organic,* if possible. Sometimes organic foods are unavailable or too expensive. Locally grown organic produce is usually reasonably priced while it's abundant and in season. Be aware that a food described as "natural" is not necessarily "organic."

- *Additive-free.* Find natural products grown and prepared without preservatives, pesticides, antibiotics, artificial colors, artificial sweeteners, and so on. Read labels!

It's good to eat a variety of foods in order to obtain a cross section of nutrients from different sources. On the other hand, research indicates that most people tend to eat the same things over and over—and this is a viable strategy for preventing overeating. If your goal is weight loss, eat a varied diet but don't feel you have to try a new recipe every night. One study revealed that people who were offered pasta in two different shapes ate more than people who were served only one shape. Variety may be the spice of life, but it also adds temptation.

Protein

We need a regular supply of protein because it's the main structural component of all our cells, which are constantly being created and renewed. Muscle, bone, tissue, and antibodies use protein for growth and repair. While your body can store energy, it has no way to store protein for a rainy day. It needs a fresh supply of quality proteins every day for cell maintenance.

Protein is made up of amino acids. "Complete" protein foods like steak and eggs include all the amino acids we need. "Incomplete" proteins, such as nuts, contain beneficial amino acids but lack one or more amino acids that the body can't synthesize. Vegans and vegetarians eat more protein from vegetable sources, which are incomplete, so they have to make sure they get all the amino acids they need.

Good sources of protein include lean meat, fish, shellfish, poultry, dairy products, eggs, legumes, nuts and seeds. To cut down on saturated fat, choose fish, lean poultry, legumes, lean cuts of meat and nonfat or low-fat dairy products, while avoiding processed foods like hot dogs or salami and anything fried.

Fats

It's true that dietary fats are high in calories, but this doesn't put all fatty foods on the forbidden list. There are healthy and unhealthy fats. The body needs healthy fats to build cells, produce hormones and maintain the oil barrier of the skin (which, among other things, helps keep germs on the outside and water on the inside). "Good" fats are helpful in keeping our blood sugar levels stable, protecting us against heart disease and satisfying our hunger. Fats also allow the body to absorb fat-soluble vitamins, such as vitamins A, D, E and K.

Saturated fats (such as the fat found in butter, cheese, cream, the skin on chicken, marbled meats, cocoa butter, and coconut, palm and palm kernel oils) are solid at room temperature. They are not good for your immune system, and they contribute to your risk of heart disease and stroke because they increase the amount of "bad" cholesterol in your blood. When you eat saturated fat, your body incorporates it into cell membranes, which become less flexible.

Monounsaturated fats (examples: olive, canola, peanut and avocado oils, and the oils in most nuts) are liquid at room temperature but start to solidify in the refrigerator. In general, they're neither "bad" nor "good" but are considered healthy when they take the place of saturated fats in your diet.

Polyunsaturated fats (examples: safflower, sesame, sunflower, corn and soybean oils) take a liquid form at room temperature and in the refrigerator. This category is a mixed bag, as it includes omega-6 fatty acids (some of which are healthier than others) as well as omega-3 fatty acids (which are very healthy).

Trans fats (or "fake fats") are created when liquid oils are artificially transformed into solid fats like hard margarine and vegetable shortening to extend their shelf life. These fats increase your "bad" cholesterol and decrease your "good" cholesterol. When you eat commercially prepared baked goods that contain trans fats, or food that has been fried in partially hydrogenated oils, your body cannot tell the difference between the trans fats and the natural fats. Even though trans fats are not a natural component of tissue, your body uses them in the building of cell membranes, where they interfere with optimal cell function.

Protein and Fats Together

Protein is often accompanied by fat. Whether this is a problem or not depends on the type of fat. A Wendy's Baconator burger has 51 grams of fat, including 22 grams of saturated fat and 2.5 grams of trans fat—all bad for you. On the other hand, 100 grams (roughly 4 ounces) of cooked wild salmon provides 2.218 grams of omega-3 fatty acids—all good for you.

When I was searching for a way to illustrate the hidden fat in food to groups that I spoke to, I came across a medical model of five pounds of fat that feels rubbery and looks, well, disgusting. People were fascinated by it! Even so, I knew I needed to find a better example, so I finally settled on a container of lard. One teaspoon of lard (saturated pork fat) equals four grams of fat. First I show the audience a McDonald's Double Quarter Pounder with Cheese. Next I ask everybody to stand up as I count out teaspoonfuls of lard and then sit down when they think I've reached the amount of saturated fat that's in the burger. One teaspoon . . . two teaspoons . . . five . . . ten . . . by now the entire audience has sat down but I'm still counting! A Double Quarter Pounder with Cheese has 48 grams of fat (or 12 teaspoons of lard). A large order of fries has 26 grams of fat (another six and a half teaspoons of lard). A 32-ounce Chocolate Triple Thick Shake contains 33 grams of fat (eight more teaspoons). The total for the burger, fries and shake comes to more than 100 grams or *26 teaspoons* of lard! By this point, the audience is really shocked. I remind them that 26 teaspoons of lard is about the equivalent of a stick of butter. Can you imagine eating a stick of butter for lunch?

Recently I read that *Men's Health* magazine had named the Aussie Cheese Fries from Outback Steakhouse as the worst food in America. The fries have bits of bacon in them and cheese sauce on top, and are served with a side of ranch dressing. They have an unbelievable 2,900 calories and 182 grams of fat—that's like eating *two* sticks of butter!

Essential Fatty Acids

We need to include essential fatty acids in our diet because the body can't synthesize them on its own. The essential fatty acids are *linoleic acid*, which is one of several omega-6 fatty acids, and *docosahexaenoic acid (DHA)*, which is one of several omega-3 fatty acids. (The remaining omega-3 and omega-6 fatty acids are, strictly speaking, not "essential" because the body has the ability to manufacture them; however, this process is inefficient and somewhat unpredictable.)

In general, we eat plenty of omega-6 fatty acids because they're readily available, but we don't get enough omega-3 fatty acids, which means we don't get enough healthy fats. This is easily remedied by eating more coldwater fish. If you prefer, you can pick up omega-3 supplements. (For more informa-tion on sources of omega-3 fatty acids, see page 242.) When you add omega-3 fatty acids to your diet, they replace the old omega-6 fats in your cell membranes. One expert refers to this as an "oil change." Studies have shown that consuming more omega-3s lowers cholesterol, reduces the risk of cardiovascular disease, boosts metabolism, helps to stabilize blood sugar, enhances nerve function and improves the healing process. Beauty experts note that increasing your intake of omega-3 fatty acids is beneficial for your skin. Eating more omega-3s can also help with arthritis conditions and diabetes, and is good for your brain as well. For all these reasons, my personal meal plan often includes an extra-large serving size of the superfood salmon.

Carbohydrates

Carbohydrates are simply sugars that are linked together. They are the primary source of fuel for our brain and muscles. During digestion, carbohydrates are broken down into glucose, which is absorbed into the bloodstream and delivered to the cells in your body, something like delivering wood for a wood-burning stove.

If you've been reading diet books, you may have picked up some unfounded ideas about

---

The Carbs to Crave

Don't let anyone set you wrong: Carbohydrates aren't *bad*, they simply must be chosen with care. Good carbs are usually nonprocessed and high in natural fiber. Include them in your diet for a maximum nutritive punch.

- **Whole fruits:**
  apples, apricots, avocados, bananas, berries, citrus fruits, cantaloupe, peaches

- **Whole grains:**
  brown rice, whole oats, and bread, cereal or crackers made from whole grain

- **Vegetables:**
  asparagus, broccoli, cabbage, cauliflower, corn, snow peas, spinach, squash, sweet potatoes

- **Legumes:**
  peas, beans, lentils

- **Nuts and seeds:**
  almonds, sunflower seeds, flaxseeds

---

carbohydrates. There is nothing "wrong" with carbohydrates, but you do need to understand which ones are good for you and which ones are not. Healthy carbohydrates, such as citrus fruits and whole grains, are rich in vitamins, minerals and dietary fiber. Refined carbohydrates are highly processed, which means most of the original nutrients and fiber have been eliminated. Table sugar, white flour, soft drinks, commercial fruit juices and other refined carbs not only add "empty calories" to your diet, but also take the place of healthy foods you could be eating instead.

Carbohydrates and Blood Sugar

It's also important to understand the relationship between carbohydrates and blood sugar. Let's say you go out to dinner to celebrate a new job. You have a fancy cocktail with fruit juice, sample the fried calamari appetizer, enjoy a fabulous pasta dish for your main course and finish up with a warm chocolate brownie topped with ice cream. This particular meal will give your body a huge hit of refined carbohydrates. The fruit juice, brownie and ice cream, which are high on the glycemic index, will quickly raise your blood sugar level and your body will have to work hard to get it back to normal. A surge of insulin will help move the sugar into your cells and extra glucose will be stored as glycogen in your liver and muscles; if the glycogen reserves in those areas are already filled up, your body will store any extra carbohydrates in the form of fat. In the future, stored glycogen and fat (in that order) can be converted back into glucose if needed.

The amount of glucose in your blood can also have an effect on your mood. When you eat refined carbohydrates, you experience a rush of energy and feel jazzed until all the glucose is used up or stored away. A low blood sugar level may follow this process, making you feel tired. Low blood sugar can also result if you get caught up in your busy day and don't stop to refuel.

When you learn how to fuel your body properly, you can sidestep these highs and lows. You can avoid seesawing blood sugar—and avoid accumulating fat—by staying away from foods that are high up on the glycemic index (such as white rice, potatoes, bread, corn) that elevate your blood sugar quickly. Instead, choose foods with a low GI value (apples, lentils, asparagus) that don't release a wave of sugar into your bloodstream.

Watch Out for Fakes!

Think of the difference between a real orange and an orange-flavored drink. The genuine orange is a wholesome food, with fiber, natural sugar and a multitude of natural plant nutrients, including vitamin C. The "fake" orange juice is now missing most of its fiber and nutrients, leaving only sugary orange-flavored water. This is a good example of why it's so important to *eat real*. You're far better off eating a whole orange, with all its pulp and natural nutrients, than drinking a glass of commercial orange juice that's been sitting on a store shelf for weeks if not months.

Choosing Real Food over Fake Food

Now that you're going to *eat real*, you will be choosing natural substances that your body can utilize instead of filling up on artificial additives and man-made chemical compounds that resemble food. To your body, there is a big difference between a box of processed potato flakes and a real mashed potato, a piece of fresh cheese and a fried mozzarella stick, or a piece of whole-grain bread and a slice of processed white bread. Always choose a natural food over a processed imitation fake food—even if the calorie content is somewhat higher. The real food is better for you.

One more reason to stick to natural foods is that we tend to eat supersized portions of the salty, sugary imitation foods because they have so little fiber. We don't feel full until it's too late.

3. Get Real

Our third fueling strategy is based on the "traffic light" approach to eating. In this approach, foods are divided into three categories: green light, yellow light and red light. I have adapted this system for the 10-Minute Total Body Breakthrough program. I've found it to be very effective because it's so easy for people to remember.

When you're driving a car, a traffic light tells you what to do:

Green says: "Go!"
Yellow tells us: "Slow down."
Red means: "Stop!"

Once you familiarize yourself with all three categories of traffic-light foods, you'll know how to make good decisions about what to eat for a life filled with energy.

Green-Light Foods– "Go!"

Green-light foods include healthy fruits and vegetables. They are plant-based (grown on trees or come from the ground) whole foods (in their natural state) that are nutrient-dense (high in vitamins, minerals and phytochemicals) and low in calories. Many of these foods are colorful—think of red peppers, green lettuce, purple grapes, pink watermelon—and they can often be eaten raw.

When eating fruits and vegetables, it's more important to get all your servings every day than to worry about the size of the orange you're about to eat or whether you should have spinach instead of Brussels sprouts. As far as I know, no one has ever developed a weight problem from eating too many of these green-light foods!

Green-Light Fruits

Apple (fresh)	1 small
Apple juice	3 ounces
Applesauce (unsweetened)	½ cup
Apricots (fresh or canned, unsweetened)	½ cup medium
Avocado (fruit)	⅛ (2 tablespoons)
Banana	½ medium
Blackberries (fresh or frozen)	½ cup
Blueberries (fresh or frozen)	½ cup
Boysenberries (fresh or frozen)	½ cup
Cantaloupe (cubed)	½ cup
Cherries (fresh)	½ cup
Cherries (canned, unsweetened)	½ cup
Cranberry juice	3 ounces
Grapefruit	½ fruit
Grapes	½ cup
Honeydew melon (cubed)	½ cup
Kiwi	1 medium
Lemon (fresh)	Any amount
Lime	Any amount
Mandarin oranges (canned segments)	⅓ cup
Mango (fresh)	⅓ fruit
Mango (frozen cubes)	½ cup
Nectarine	1
Orange	1 small
Orange juice	⅓ cup
Papaya	1 small
Papaya (frozen cubes)	½ cup
Peach	½
Peach halves (canned, unsweetened)	⅛ cup
Pear	½ small
Pear halves (canned, unsweetened)	2
Pineapple	½ cup
Pineapple (canned in its own juice)	⅓ cup chunks
Plum	1 small
Prunes	2
Raisins	1 mini-box (25 raisins)
Raspberries (fresh or frozen)	½ cup
Strawberries	1 cup
Tangerine	1 small
Watermelon (cubed)	1 cup

Green-Light Vegetables

Asparagus	1½ cups, cooked
Broccoli	1 cup, cooked
Brussels sprouts	1 cup, cooked
Cabbage	2 cups, cooked
Carrots	1 cup, cooked
Cauliflower	2 cups, cooked
Eggplant	2 cups, cooked
Lettuce	Unlimited
Mushrooms	2 cups, raw
Onions	1 cup, raw; ¾ cup, cooked
Peas	½ cup raw
Peppers	2 cups, raw; 1 cup, cooked
Radishes	2 cups, raw
Snow peas	1½ cups, raw
Spinach	1½ cups, cooked
Tomatoes	2 cups, fresh; 1½ cups, canned; ¼ cup, paste

Yellow-Light Foods– "Slow Down"

Yellow-light foods have more calories (in the form of protein, carbohydrate or fat) than green-light foods, so serving sizes become more important. You don't have to count calories, but do keep an eye on how much you eat. Yellow-light foods are divided into complex carbohydrates (including whole grains, starches and legumes) and proteins. Items that are higher in carbohydrates have smaller serving sizes. For example, a medium baked potato counts as one serving. In general, an appropriate serving of protein is about the size of a deck of cards or the palm of your hand. Exceptions include firm cheeses (eat less, because of the saturated fat content) and salmon (go ahead—eat more!).

Going Nuts

Nuts went out of fashion when people became afraid of their fat content. Happily, a lot has been learned about their health benefits and—in moderation—they're back on the menu.

You can eat nuts plain or enjoy them in your meals. I recommend tossing some nuts into your yogurt, oatmeal or breakfast cereal, or mixing a handful into your next salad or stir-fry. Nut butters are always delicious, and the healthy fats they contain can bring down the GI values of foods like bread and crackers when you eat them together. You also can use nut butters in baking (anyone for peanut butter cookies?) or gourmet cooking (for example, grilled salmon with Asian peanut sauce). I make my own hummus using a can of chickpeas, fresh garlic, extra-virgin olive oil, lemon juice and a couple of tablespoons of peanut butter or sesame tahini.

Overall, nuts are a good source of protein and are good for your heart—they have no cholesterol and are high in monounsaturated fats. Research shows that people who eat nuts at least twice a week are less likely to gain weight than people who avoid nuts. A meta-analysis of several studies showed that people who eat nuts at least four times a week have a 37% lower risk of coronary heart disease than people who seldom eat nuts. Moreover, each additional serving of nuts further reduces the risk.

Almonds. These nuts are unusually high in vitamin E and also contain helpful amounts of manganese (involved in bone formation and in metabolizing protein, fats and carbohydrates) and magnesium (good for healthy bones and keeping nerves relaxed). Twenty different antioxidants have been identified in the dark skins of almonds, and the flavonoids in the skins work together with the vitamin E in the almond meat to enhance the resistance of LDL cholesterol to oxidation. As part of a heart-healthy diet, almonds have been shown to reduce cholesterol levels as much as some cholesterol-lowering drugs and to lower the risk of gaining weight; in fact, eating almonds as part of a low-calorie diet may actually help you lose weight. One ounce of almonds has 163 calories and 6 grams of protein.

Cashews. These nuts have a lower fat content than most other nuts. About 75% of the unsaturated fat in cashews is oleic acid, the same heart-healthy fat found in olive oil. One ounce of raw cashews has 155 calories and 5 grams of protein, plus helpful

Yellow-Light Carbohydrates

Bagel, whole-grain	½
Bread, whole-grain	1 regular slice
Brown rice	⅓ cup, cooked
Cereal, whole-grain	½ cup
Crackers, whole-wheat	4
Lentils	½ cup, cooked
Oats, old-fashioned	¾ cup, cooked
Pasta, whole-wheat	½ cup, cooked
Potato	1 small, cooked
Rice cakes, plain	3
Sweet potato	½ cup, cooked
Tortilla, whole-wheat	1 6"

Yellow-Light Proteins/Fats

Almonds (whole)	1 ounce, raw
Beef (lean)	3 ounces, cooked
Cashews	1 ounce
Cheese (nonfat)	3 ounces
Chicken (breast, skinless)	3 ounces (½ breast), cooked
Cod (Atlantic)	3–4 ounces
Cottage cheese (low-fat or nonfat)	1 cup
Eggs	2 (or 1½ cups egg whites)
Flaxseed	2 tablespoons
Haddock	3–4 ounces
Halibut	3–4 ounces
Milk (nonfat)	2 cups
Peanuts (unsweetened)	1 ounce
Peanut butter (all natural)	1½ tablespoons
Salmon	4–6 ounces, cooked
Trout	4 ounces, cooked
Tuna (canned, packed in water)	¾ can
Turkey (sliced, deli style)	4 slices
Walnuts	1 ounce
Yogurt, low-fat	1 cup

amounts of manganese and magnesium. Cashews, like other nuts, should be part of any weight-loss or weight-maintenance diet.

Walnuts. One ounce of raw walnuts has 183 calories, 4 grams of protein and a good amount of manganese. Walnuts are also a good source of omega-3 fatty acids, which have a huge range of health benefits. Among other things, omega-3s are anti-inflammatory and combat chronic illnesses

Peanuts and the French Paradox

Technically a peanut is a legume, not a nut. One ounce of peanuts has 159 calories and 7 grams of protein, plus helpful amounts of manganese and folate. Peanuts are a good source of heart-healthy monounsaturated fats. As an added bonus, they contain small amounts of resveratrol, a plant compound also found in red wine, grapes, blueberries and cranberries. In the lab, resveratrol has increased blood flow to the brain and has demonstrated anti-inflammatory and anticancer properties. It also has been associated with extending the lifespan of yeast, worms, fruit flies and fish. It is not known whether resveratrol can extend the human lifespan, but some people believe resveratrol may help explain "the French paradox"—the fact that French people can smoke and eat fabulous foods containing saturated fats such as brie and pâté without getting fat or developing heart disease.

like asthma and arthritis; they enhance circulation and protect against heart disease; they promote better cognitive function and combat depression; they protect against bone loss; and they support the immune system.

Walnuts also contain l-arginine, an amino acid that the body converts into nitric oxide, which helps blood vessels relax. This means walnuts are especially beneficial for people who are interested in controlling their blood pressure. Researchers found that when people ate a high-fat meal that included walnuts, their blood circulation increased, and that the same meal without the walnuts caused a decrease in blood flow. The FDA has formally approved the health claim that eating 1.5 ounces of walnuts per day as part of a diet low in saturated fat and cholesterol may reduce the risk of heart disease. As if all this were not enough, walnuts also lower cholesterol and are high in antioxidants—including melatonin, produced in the human body as the "sleep hormone."

Red-Light Foods– "Stop!"

Red-light foods are those you will want to stop and think about before eating. Ask yourself: "Is this what I need right now?" "Can my body use this food in a healthy way?" "If I eat this now, am I going to be sorry later?" "Is there an alternative that would be better for me?" "Could I eat just a small portion—then stop?" These foods may have lots of calories but few nutrients (examples: alcohol, cookies, doughnuts), lots of saturated fat, hydrogenated oils or trans fats (margarine, salad dressing, hot dogs, fried foods) and lots of sugar (candy, soda, ice cream). They also have artificial sweeteners, additives and preservatives.

In my experience, people do not like being told what they cannot eat. I never forbid my clients to eat anything, because this turns many people into two-year-olds. If they think they may never again have a Big Mac, the usual reaction is "Who says I can't?" Outlawing certain foods also condemns people to failure. When people slip (which we all do sometimes), they feel guilty. Instead of picking themselves up and starting over, they give up altogether or maybe even go on to do something worse. They feel they can't succeed at being perfect, so why bother trying?

Studies show that the human brain needs to work with positives. A "can-do" message gives the brain something concrete on which to focus, whereas being negative gives the brain nothing to work with. For example, when people heard the old campaign "Don't drink and drive," their brains could not grasp the non-message of *not* doing something. So the advice their brains took away was "Drink and drive." The new slogan is "Drink responsibly," which gives the brain an action on which to focus, and people a positive behavior to follow. In terms of eating, if you're told that under *no* circumstances should you ever, *ever* have another cookie for the rest of your life, what's the first thing you want? Your brain is looking for something concrete, so the very thing you're *not* supposed to think about becomes the focus of your attention. Given such restrictions, food becomes either "good" or "bad," and here's the kicker: This way of thinking ultimately leaves us feeling either good or bad about ourselves, based upon what we eat.

When it comes to fueling for life, I teach people what they *can* enjoy. In other words, if a dollop of sour cream, a few bacon bits or a sprinkle of Parmesan cheese makes the difference between "edible" and "inedible" for you, I'd rather have you eat these small amounts of red-light foods and stay within healthy guidelines than give up on healthy eating altogether. If you've slathered ketchup on your food all your life, use smaller and smaller amounts until one fine day you realize that ketchup doesn't really enhance the taste of the healthy whole foods you're eating. I say, "Focus on the best and decrease the rest."

The occasional cookie does not represent failure. I tell all my clients they can eat whatever they want. They have complete freedom to choose. Then my goal is to educate them about making the best possible choices about when and what to eat. After their hunger is satisfied and their need for essential nutrients is met with green-light and yellow-light foods, making wise decisions about red-light foods is much easier.

Keep It Real

Small amounts of red-light foods that are natural and preferably organic are better for you than cheap imitations filled with corn syrup, dyes and chemical additives. I would much rather have you eat a small amount of all-natural, sugar-free fruit preserves on your toast than that "fruit spread" I mentioned earlier.

Choose a Small Amount of This Real Food . . .	Instead of This Fake Food
100% maple syrup	Imitation pancake syrup
Genuine whipped cream	Frozen or aerosol dessert topping
Milk	Nondairy creamer
Frozen yogurt with genuine yogurt cultures	Soft-serve imitation frozen yogurt
Fresh cooked pasta with a sprinkle of Parmesan	Macaroni and cheese from a box
A few almonds, raisins and dark chocolate morsels	Commercial "trail mix"

How to Build a Healthy Meal

Now for the fun part: fueling at the speed of life! My "get real" 4•3•2•1 approach to meal planning is flexible and fast. It helps you focus on eating healthy foods in the correct amounts without counting points or playing any calorie games. It's easier when you're at home and have your favorite foods on hand, but the same principles apply wherever you are. Whether you're grabbing a quick breakfast in the kitchen or going out for dinner to an "all you can eat" buffet, now you will know exactly what to do.

You want to eat a majority of green-light foods, so ideally every meal, including breakfast, should feature an array of fruits and vegetables. Yellow-light carbohydrates will provide fiber and essential nutrients and will help to regulate your blood sugar level. The protein/fat portion of your meal is the smallest part.

The 4•3•2•1 Portion Plate

To figure out your portions, picture your plate as a pie that has been cut in half with one of the halves cut into thirds. Then follow the 4•3•2•1 format:

4 ounces of water before and after your meal

Water is the ultimate energy beverage. Drinking 4 ounces (half a cup) of water *before* each meal and snack helps to suppress your appetite. It has also been found that if you drink water *after* your meal, you're free to concentrate on chewing your food *during* the meal, which aids digestion. But don't limit yourself—drink as much water as you can throughout the day.

3 servings of green-light fruits and vegetables

Your goal is to fill half your plate with three servings of green-light fruits and vegetables. If weight loss is your goal, go easy on the fruits, because they have more sugar. However, this is not a diet! I don't want you to get out your calorie counter to figure out the difference in calories between apple and zucchini, since both are good for you.

2 servings of yellow-light healthy carbohydrates

Fill two-thirds of the other side of your plate with two servings of yellow-light starches and whole grains. Remember, one serving of carbohydrate would be *two* slices of commercial diet bread (not the best choice, but sometimes that's all there is) or *one* slice of hearty whole-grain bread (much better for you, but also heavier).

1 serving of yellow-light protein/fat

The remaining third of your plate is for protein, which usually has a certain amount of fat in it. An appropriate serving of yellow-light protein, such as lean beef or half a skinless chicken breast, is 3 or 4 ounces.

Here's how your plate should look:*

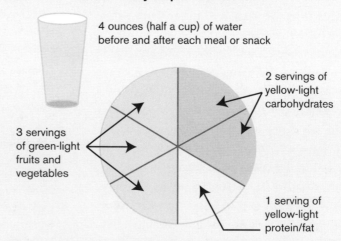

4 ounces (half a cup) of water before and after each meal or snack

2 servings of yellow-light carbohydrates

3 servings of green-light fruits and vegetables

1 serving of yellow-light protein/fat

* In the near future, it's likely that you'll be able to know more about your genetic predispositions and metabolism. When that happens, meal servings will undoubtedly be modified to meet your specific needs and goals.

Building a 4·3·2·1 Snack

To construct a healthy snack, start with a serving of a yellow-light protein, then add *either* a green-light fruit/vegetable *or* a yellow-light carbohydrate. Snacks have fewer servings overall than meals, but the serving sizes remain the same. This makes snack portions easy to remember.

Eating Out

Americans love their fast food, and many of my clients grab meals on the run. Now that you'll be eating more nutritious foods, you'll want to find ways to make a fast switch to healthier meals. For example, instead of a cheeseburger with special sauce, choose a veggie burger or a small burger on a whole-grain bun with lettuce, tomato and pickle. And forget the pizza with salami, sausage or pepperoni—the pizza with a whole-wheat crust and half the cheese or the vegetarian pizza with just the whole-wheat crust is the way to go.

Many websites offer lists of the "least terrible" choices from the menus at a variety of fast-food chains. To take the guesswork out of what you *think* you're putting into your body, look for a site that gives total calories, percentage of fat, grams of protein and carbohydrate content of each food selection.

Snack Time

Option #1

Combine one serving of a green-light fruit or vegetable with a serving of yellow-light protein/fat. Here are some ideas:

Apple *with* all-natural peanut butter	
Banana *with* plain, low-fat or nonfat yogurt	
Blueberries *with* low-fat or nonfat cottage cheese	
Peach *with* almonds	
Carrots *with* turkey	

Option #2

Combine one serving of yellow-light carbohydrate with a snack-size serving of yellow-light protein/fat. Some ideas:

Rice cake *with* edamame (soybeans)	
1/2 whole-grain bagel *with* tuna, canned, in water	
1 slice whole-grain bread *with* hard-boiled egg	
Whole-grain cereal *with* low-fat or nonfat milk	
Whole-wheat crackers *with* cheese	
Whole-wheat or corn tortilla *with* chicken	

Most full-service restaurants offer heart-healthy menu options, so getting the right foods should not be difficult. If one particular restaurant serves only entrées that are fried, cooked in butter or piled high with cheese, find a different one! To learn more about smart choices, go to www.4321fitness.com.

Nutrition at the Speed of Life

The healthiest and best way to lose excess body fat and get in top shape is to do your 10-minute workouts and to eat five or six times a day, getting the most nutrients possible with the fewest calories. But fueling your body in the right balance five or six times a day can seem like a daunting task. Even with the best of intentions, taking the time and energy to select and prepare a well-balanced meal or snack with healthy and real ingredients just doesn't always happen.

Choosing a Multivitamin Supplement

Vitamins, minerals, phytochemicals and other trace nutrients are necessary in forming new tissues, completing chemical reactions, and keeping your eyes, skin, hair, teeth, bones and the trillions of cells throughout your body functioning effectively. You also can help your body stay healthy by maximizing your intake of antioxidants, which help your body combat free radicals. A natural by-product of exercise, exposure to toxins, sun exposure, and so on, free radicals cause cellular damage that accumulates until bigger problems appear. They're associated with a wide variety of age-related disorders, including cancer, macular degeneration, heart disease and Parkinson's disease, and also cause age-related changes in the skin that contribute to wrinkles and sagging. Happily, fat- and water-soluble antioxidants do a good job of fighting these problems.

Eating a wide variety of unprocessed foods is the best way to ensure you get all the vitamins, minerals, antioxidants and phytochemicals your body needs every day. Unfortunately, most of us do not consume all the foods necessary to meet our body's needs. Also, each one of us is biochemically unique, which means some people just naturally have a greater need for certain nutrients than other people.

Because of our biochemical individuality, hectic lifestyles, poor eating habits and food sources that are less than optimal, plus our exposure to the hazards of modern life, most of us have some kind of nutrient insufficiency that can compromise our energy level, vitality, fitness and health. You don't need to have an actual deficiency to feel the effects of low levels of a nutrient.

You can help provide your body with what it needs by using a natural vitamin/mineral supplement bought from a reputable company. A good general-purpose supplement will include a wide variety of nutrients in the correct doses. Look for one that includes antioxidants like vitamins A, C and E. In your vitamin/mineral supplement, also look for vitamins D, K, B_6, and B_{12}, thiamin, pantothenic acid, riboflavin, niacin, folic acid, biotin, calcium, magnesium, phosphorus, iodine, iron, copper, molybdenum, chromium, manganese, zinc and selenium.

Vitamin/mineral supplements are available at health food stores, grocery stores, independent supplement distributors, vitamin shops, online, or at many drugstores. But before you choose one, be aware that all vitamins are not the same. Look for companies that use organic farming practices, extensive product research and first-rate manufacturing practices and provide extensive quality assurance.

Protein Bars, Shakes and Smoothies

The good news is that a few reputable health and nutrition companies are producing high-tech, high-quality protein bars and drinks containing the proper balance of nutrients to help you fuel your body and mind throughout the day. I use these items for snacks and/or meals when I'm on the run and need some fast fueling. They can be carried anywhere, and they take the guesswork out of eating right. Many of our superstar clients use these foods to help them eat every three hours while controlling their calories. Of course, protein bars and drinks are meant to be supplements, not substitutes for a healthy diet, and you still need to provide your body with a variety of natural whole foods, but these items are great for those times when:

- You're in a rush in the morning and there's no time to fix breakfast.

- You're tempted to skip a meal because you're too busy.

- You're so hungry that you're about to grab a red-light food.

- You're going to be working out soon and your muscles need energy.

- You just finished a workout and your muscles need protein.

There are hundreds of products to choose from, but all you need for your new fitness program is some protein powder to make a nutritious protein smoothie and possibly some protein bars or ready-made shakes to have on hand when you're in a hurry. I recommend whey protein isolate powder (go to www.4321fitness .com to learn about quality protein supplements).

The Basic 4•3•2•1 Protein Smoothie Recipe

This smoothie may be prepared the night before and refrigerated until breakfast. Or you can put the ingredients in the glass pitcher of the blender the night before, place the pitcher in your refrigerator and process the smoothie in the morning.

- *4 ounces (half a cup) nonfat milk*
- *3 ounces (6 tablespoons) protein powder*
- *2 servings fresh or frozen fruit (see page 60 for serving sizes)*
- *1 ounce raw skin-on almonds (not roasted, not salted)*

Directions

1. Place milk and almonds in the blender. Process until smooth and creamy, with no nut fragments.
2. Add fruit in small pieces and process again.
3. Add protein powder and process until smooth.
4. Enjoy!

Smoothie Variations

- Use 4 ounces of orange juice instead of milk.
- If you're using fresh fruit, add 3 or 4 ice cubes to the blender for a cooler, more refreshing drink.

- If you prefer your smoothies on the sweet side, add honey. (Be aware that this will increase the total number of calories.)
- Add a few drops of vanilla, almond or coconut extract for flavoring.
- For an extra-creamy smoothie, add half a cup of fruit or vanilla yogurt, preferably low-fat and low-sugar. (This will add roughly 50 calories—not that we're counting!)
- Use a different kind of nut. Raw cashew pieces blend particularly well and are nutritionally similar to almonds.

The 4•3•2•1 Protein Smoothie

Whether you're running late for breakfast, need some protein just to help build your muscles after a workout, or want an afternoon snack and are about to reach for last night's dessert, whip up a smoothie before you do anything you might regret. To make sure you have a way to fuel your body correctly in any situation, I developed the 4•3•2•1 Protein Smoothie—a homemade super smoothie that gives you a nutritious meal in a glass in no time flat.

In this one satisfying and delicious drink, with only 390 calories, you get a good supply of protein (30.5 grams) for building and repairing your tissues, healthy fats (14 grams) for creating cell membranes, carbohydrates (35 grams, depending on fruit selected) for burning for energy, and fiber (6.25 grams) for your gastrointestinal tract, plus calcium for your bones, vitamins, minerals and antioxidants (depending on the fruit you use). If you feel that the 4•3•2•1 Protein Smoothie has too many calories for your diet plan, use less protein powder and/or fewer nuts, or divide the basic smoothie in half and use it for two snacks.

Berry Blast Smoothie

- *4 ounces nonfat milk*
- *4 ounces plain yogurt*
- *3 ounces vanilla-flavored protein powder*
- *2 servings of mixed berries (1 cup each of strawberries and/or blueberries, raspberries and blackberries)*
- *1 ounce raw almonds*

Variation: Use half a cup of berries and half a banana.

Almond Apple Pie Smoothie

- *4 ounces nonfat milk*
- *3 ounces vanilla-flavored protein powder*
- *2 servings of fruit: 1 small apple, 3 ounces apple juice*
- *1 ounce raw almonds*
- *Add ¼ teaspoon cinnamon and a dash of nutmeg.*

Sweeten to taste.
Variation: Add 4 ounces vanilla yogurt.

Chocolate Raspberry Smoothie

- *4 ounces nonfat milk*
- *3 ounces chocolate-flavored protein powder*
- *2 servings of fruit: 1 cup fresh or frozen raspberries*
- *1 ounce raw almonds*

Sweeten to taste.
Variation: Use cherries instead of raspberries.

Orange Peach Mango Smoothie

- *4 ounces orange juice*
- *3 ounces vanilla-flavored protein powder*
- *2 servings of fruit: ½ cup peaches and ½ cup mangoes*
- *1 ounce raw almonds*

Sweeten to taste.
Variation: Use raw cashew pieces instead of almonds.

Melon Milk Smoothie

- *4 ounces nonfat milk*
- *3 ounces vanilla-flavored protein powder*
- *2 servings of fruit: 2 cups watermelon*
- *1 ounce raw almonds*

Sweeten to taste.
Variation: Use honeydew or cantaloupe.

When it comes to protein drinks, there's no such thing as a "one size fits all" recipe. Experiment with different ingredients and different serving sizes until you find what works for you. For even more super Smoothie recipes, go to www.4321fitness.com.

Are You Ready to Change Your Life?

The 10-Minute Total Body Breakthrough program provides you with everything you need for success. Your job now is to follow the daily instructions, learn how to do the 10-minute workouts and fuel your body in a healthy way. Then, stand back! Your increased fitness will change every area of your life.

By now, you're probably saying "Okay, Sean, I get it!" Believe me, I'm as eager as you are to have you start living the 4•3•2•1 program . . . now! And remember, I'm your coach, here to take you through the same process my personal training clients go through. If you stick with me—identifying your readiness to change, determining your personal barriers, setting personal goals, assessing your personal fitness level—you will succeed. If you're not convinced, take a peek at Chapter 11, where you'll find more of my 4•3•2•1 successes.

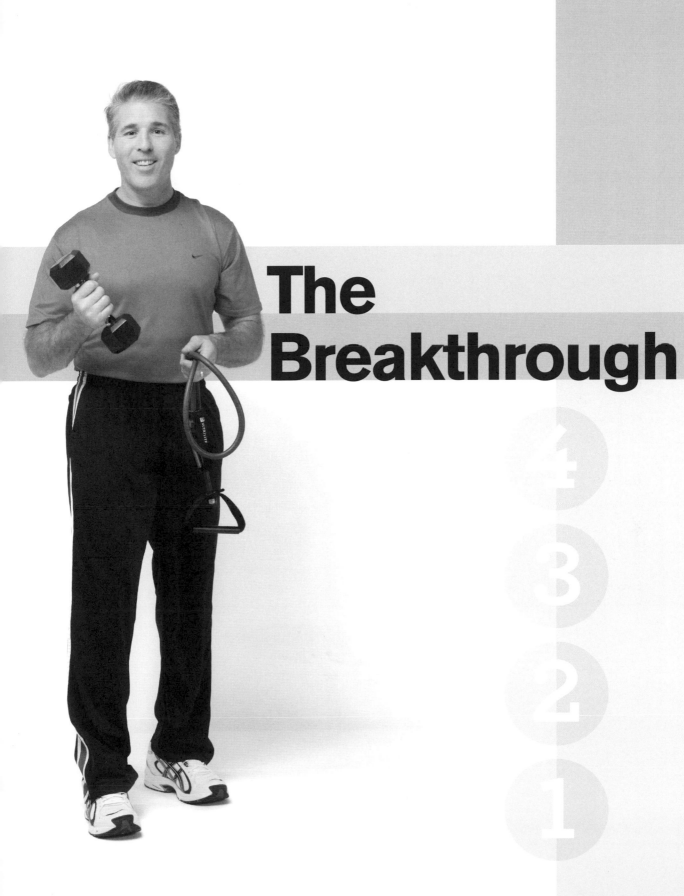

The
Breakthrough

4
3
2
1

chapter 6

Ready, Set . . . Go!

It's Time to Take Action

I once sat on a plane next to a psychotherapist who used an interesting expression as we talked about health and fitness. She said, "Emotions are the tail over the fence." What she meant was: First you change your behavior, and then your emotions follow. When you behave as if you have no fear, you eventually become fearless. When you act in a loving manner, real love can grow. When you exercise, eat the right foods and take time for renewal and reflection, you create an ongoing desire for good health. In other words, you don't have to love every minute of your new fitness program, but give it a chance and eventually you will!

Don't let past failures stand in your way. This is a totally new approach to exercise, both fast and fun. And because it's a proven program, based on the latest scientific breakthroughs, you can have full confidence that it will work.

The Stages of Change

Even the most positive changes take us away from our familiar habits and routines and out of our comfort zone. James Prochaska, author of *Changing for Good,* has made a science of studying people who successfully make significant changes. He has identified six steps in his "stages of change" model. I have adapted them to your personal journey into fitness.

Stage 1: Pre-contemplation
"I don't need to change."

During Stage 1, you feel you have no control over the problem, and you're not even thinking about making any changes. This stage is characterized by defensive, counterproductive behavior like blaming, denial and rationalizing. By ignoring or minimizing the problem, you can protect your current way of life and spare yourself the effort or discomfort of change. Most people in this stage would not bother to read a fitness book.

You can make positive use of this stage by identifying the common defenses that let you keep your awareness of the problem at bay. Recognizing your defenses will move you closer to the next stage.

Stage 2: Contemplation
"I'm thinking about maybe changing."

During this stage, you begin to think about the possibility of making positive changes. This stage is characterized by an awareness of the problem along with behavior that doesn't move you forward, such as wishful thinking, waiting for a magic cure and collecting data. You know you should do something, but you don't want to change your routine, so you procrastinate. You may even set a date, but you keep postponing it.

You can make positive use of this stage by taking a good look at the consequences of the way you live now, by thinking about the benefits of changing and by honestly examining your barriers to change. Focusing on the future encourages you to become a problem solver rather than a problem dweller.

Because you're reading this book, I'm guessing that right now you're in Stage 2. You know you need to change, and you're looking for the best way to make your fitness dreams a reality. Look no further: The 10-Minute Total Body Breakthrough program does everything for you but the actual exercises!

Stage 3: Preparation
"I'm planning on making a change."

By the time you reach this point, making a change has become a priority for you. This stage is for planning, like a dress rehearsal for the real performance, and is characterized by announcing your intention to others, determining your motivation (your deepest "why"), considering your options, setting appropriate goals and establishing the steps you'll take to make your transformation. You will begin to ask yourself questions such as: Where and when will I exercise? What do I need to organize before I get started? What healthy foods should I have on hand? What sensible snacks will work for me? Do I need to buy exercise clothes, a mini-cooler, a blender or a journal? This book has simplified Stage 3 for you—each detail of your fitness program is covered in the daily instructions starting on page 236.

Stage 4: Action
"I'm changing!"

Now it's time to "just do it." Set a date and get started. You already have a good plan; now you need to supply confidence, optimism, determination, focus and hard work. You can help yourself by keeping yourself motivated. Leave yourself notes; put a picture of yourself or your family on the refrigerator; don't forget your positive affirmations. A supportive environment is very helpful, so get others involved in your success. Remember your connections!

Some people jump directly to Stage 4 without going through the earlier stages, but this usually doesn't work. Despite their enthusiasm, they most likely will revert until they work through the necessary processes that come before Action.

This stage is characterized by new thoughts and

behaviors. Eventually your new workout routines and food choices will become familiar. During this learning stage, keep in mind that your goal is not short-term gratification but lifelong success. This book will keep you focused and will provide activities to speed your transformation mentally, physically, spiritually and in terms of your relationships.

Stage 5: Maintenance
"Now I want to stay this way."

Generally this stage arrives after about three to six months of changed behavior at Stage 4. The good news is that now you know you can do all the right things to live a healthy lifestyle. The bad news is that challenges are inevitable. You may hit a plateau, you may be vulnerable to temptation or you may get off track because of illness. You can make positive use of this stage by perfecting your technique, learning new exercises and challenging yourself with new fitness goals. Continue to seek support, even though the novelty has worn off, and stay positive.

Stage 6: Termination
"I did it! What's next?"

The name of this stage needs some explaining. It means you can now wrap up this particular change cycle. You no longer have to make an effort to be successful, because you've established healthy habits.

By continuing to do new things, you will continue to create new neural pathways in your brain. New pathways mean new connections and new possibilities. Sometimes you may backtrack a step or two. Just remember that relapsing is better than not making any changes at all! Prochaska says, "The only mistake you can make is to give up on yourself."

What Are Your Barriers?

As you get ready to begin your new fitness regimen, you need to identify the roadblocks that have been keeping you from making positive changes. The program is designed to *break through* these stubborn barriers—and I've heard them all!

Which barrier(s) below have prevented positive changes in your life?

☐ **"I don't have time."** *Solution:* The 4•3•2•1 program will help you get fit using workouts that last just 10 minutes.

☐ **"Exercise is too boring."** *Solution:* Using the different 10-minute workouts, you'll become fit without spending hours on the treadmill or endlessly repeating the same exercise regimen. Using the different workouts, you can create hundreds of different routines.

☐ **"I'm too tired after work."** *Solution:* With a workout that lasts just 10 minutes, you don't have to wait until evening to exercise. Plus, once you get started on your new fitness regimen, you'll have more energy all day.

☐ **"I'm too old."** *Solution:* Exercise is beneficial for people of all ages, sizes and fitness levels. In one strength-training study, the average age of the participants was 92!

☐ **"I'm sick."** *Solution:* Moderate exercise is appropriate for people with chronic illnesses because it enhances circulation, builds strength and boosts the immune system.

☐ **"I have a bad back (knee, elbow)."** *Solution:* I have helped hundreds of people just like you to become fit and limber.

☐ **"Exercising is too expensive."** *Solution:* You can buy a few items for a home exercise area for under $50 (see pages 134–136). If you belong to a gym, you'll get more for your money if you use the 10-minute workouts.

☐ **"Women aren't supposed to lift weights."** *Solution:* Women of all ages and fitness levels can, and do, lift weights. With the 10-minute workouts, you won't develop bulky muscles.

☐ **"I don't like exercising around other people."** *Solution:* If you prefer to sweat by yourself, do your workouts at home or outdoors.

☐ **"I don't like exercising alone."** *Solution:* If you're a social exerciser, grab a friend, start a 10-Minute Total Body Breakthrough group or go to the gym.

☐ **"I'll get to it soon, I promise!"** *Solution:* No more procrastinating. Success is now within your reach. Just set the date that will mark the beginning of your new healthy life.

How to Set S.M.A.R.T. Goals

Some people say they can't get started on a fitness regimen unless they're feeling fired up. If you're already feeling enthusiastic, that's great. It will make your new beginning that much easier. But you might want to look at it the Yogi Berra way. "You've got to be very careful if you don't know where you're going," he once said, "because you might not get there." I'm fairly certain what he meant is: The only way to make certain progress is to have a goal. "S.M.A.R.T. goals" is a popular term in management circles that can be easily adapted to your journey of transformation. Choose goals that are:

Specific. Precisely what do you want to accomplish? Weight reduction? Better muscle tone? Stress reduction? Improved sports performance? What exactly will be different? How will you know when you have achieved success?

Measurable. The only way to know if you have accomplished anything is to pick a goal that can be measured. Do you want to lose inches? Drop pounds? Complete a certain number of repetitions? Decide on the level of improvement you want to accomplish.

Action. Choose a goal that has steps you can take for success. Make your goal positive and specific. A negative and/or vague goal—for example, "I don't want to be depressed anymore"—doesn't tell you what you can do to fix the problem.

Realistic. A goal that is too lofty will lead to disillusionment. If you have a giant long-term goal, break it down into reasonable short-term goals that you can achieve and celebrate. This will give you a much-needed sense of accomplishment from day to day and week to week. Don't make any plans that depend on doing something that will never happen. If you live in Iowa, don't plan to surf. If you hate to jog, don't buy a treadmill.

Timed. For each goal, set a target date by which you will accomplish it. Challenge yourself, but be realistic as well. If you choose it correctly, this date will be a strong motivating factor for you. Use it to keep yourself on track.

Making It Work: You Can Do It!

When I first explain a 10-minute workout, people usually say, "Okay, I can do that." The amount of time is manageable, and the exercises can be adapted to suit any fitness level. The whole process is broken down into small steps that anyone can handle, so that progress can be measured each day.

Research shows that people do better when they feel optimistic about their chance of success. This may seem like a blinding flash of the obvious, but it has many implications, particularly because the reverse is also true. When people believe they cannot be successful, they aren't—whether or not their belief was well founded. Dr. Albert Bandura called this concept "self-efficacy," and he said an individual's self-efficacy is a greater predictor of success than whether or not it objectively appears likely that someone will be successful. Willpower is not the most important factor, and brains do not guarantee success. They key element to success is confidence.

Some days will be better than others. Just continue to focus on what you did well, and soon enough you will see an increase in both your confidence and momentum. Give yourself time. It may not happen right away, but ultimately, if you stay the course, you will reach your desired destination. Focus on the process, and the results will come.

Baby Steps

One of the best ways to increase your self-efficacy is to take small, achievable steps and to deliberately create scenarios in which you can succeed. This helps explain why the 10-Minute Total Body Breakthrough is so effective. Success begets success.

Take a look at successful athletes, musicians or businesspeople. How do they explain their success or mastery? Did it happen overnight? We may think it came quickly, but most likely they spent day in and day out practicing, working and moving one inch closer until they "suddenly" became famous. Similarly, individuals who are financially successful usually make regular investments and over time see dramatic compounding effects upon their personal wealth.

The Japanese have a term, *kaizen,* that roughly translates as "continuous incremental improvement." They apply this concept to different situations, including workplace efficiency. Here at home, we have the story of the tortoise and the hare and, more recently, two books: one by John Trent, called *The 2-Degree Difference: How Little Things Can Change Everything,* and another by Robert Maurer, Ph.D., called *One Small Step Can Change Your Life.* In every example, the key to success goes not to the swift but to the persistent. When we make "inch by inch" investments in our bodies, relationships and spiritual lives, eventually we begin to reap significant benefits. While it might seem unfamiliar and frustrating to take this approach in a fast-paced society where much is made of sudden, dramatic change, the one-step-at-a-time approach is a proven method to guarantee your success. I often tell my kids that good things take time—for example, it took nine months to make each of them!

Plan for Success– Every Day

The next two sections, *plan for success* and *track your progress,* are closely related. They're like a one-two punch that will knock out your old habits and let you replace them with new, healthy behaviors. The following tips will help you plan for success.

- **Plan your exercise sessions.** At the beginning of your week, sit down with your calendar and block out the exact times you will exercise. Schedule at least three 10-minute 4•3•2•1 workouts and three 10-minute blocks of time for general exercise. Check the daily instructions for the week, as they will have recommendations for each day. Treat your exercise like any other important appointment. Don't rely on fitting in your workouts "whenever," and don't let any sudden turn of events push your exercise sessions off your calendar. Your commitment to exercising must be absolute!

- **Plan to exercise in the morning whenever possible.** Exercising first thing in the morning has the added benefit of giving you a metabolic boost for the whole day. It also appears to help with compliance. Many of my clients say they exercise in the morning in order to make sure they get it done. If you don't exercise first thing, something is likely to come up that will make taking even just 10 minutes for exercise more difficult.

- **Plan your meals and snacks.** It's a good idea to plan what you're going to eat, instead of hoping the right food will appear at the right time. This simple step will help your success dramatically. When you anticipate your meals for the week, you'll be sure to buy the right groceries, which avoids putting you in the position of having to eat the wrong foods because you're starving

Stay in the Moment

Focusing on everything you need to accomplish in order to become fit can be overwhelming if you don't think in terms of one step at a time. An excellent anti-stress technique is to breathe deeply and remind yourself that, at this particular moment, you are okay. You're in one piece. You're breathing. For this moment, that's all you need. Keep your eyes closed, if you wish. After your anxiety about the big picture passes, you will open your eyes and handle your immediate challenge with new clarity.

and the cupboard is bare. Also, when you know you have healthy items at home, you're less vulnerable to temptations like unscheduled stops for fast food. At the beginning of each week, check to see if there are any tricky situations coming up, such as a long conference, a late dinner date, a cocktail party or big celebration. Be prepared with healthy snacks, bottled water or whatever else you need to stay on track.

■ **Write down your goals.** There is something extremely powerful in writing down your plans, then checking them off one by one as you successfully complete them. With each item checked, you gain a sense of confidence in your ability to make things happen and ultimately move closer to your long-term goals. With this in mind, take a moment each morning to write down your exercise goals for the day. Planning your priorities before life gets going is one of the easiest and most effective steps you can take to ensure your transformation.

Track Your Progress

When it comes to weight loss, study after study indicates that individuals who track their behavior—how much they exercise, what they eat, and so on—lose significantly more weight than those who do not. Also, researchers found that people who continue to track their behavior over the long term maintain their weight loss much more successfully than those who do not. Unfortunately, researchers also discovered that, for most of us, tracking is very difficult. We just don't like to do it! In multiple studies, participants who were asked to monitor their food intake or exercise habits kept their records for less than half the necessary time of the study. And they even had counselors to remind them.

So we have a dilemma. Tracking is essential for our transformation, but few of us like to do it. Your way out of this dilemma is to:

1. Accept that tracking your progress will help you over the long term, and

2. Figure out a method that will work for you personally. People who become effective at tracking their behavior understand why it's important to do so, and they treat it as a skill they can learn to master. There is no "standard" formula or procedure; the best tracking system is the one that you will use.

The daily instructions in Chapter 10 remind you to take a few moments every night to reflect on your day. At a minimum, write a few thoughts in the journal space provided. Tracking your steps toward your ultimate transformation is one of the single most effective and essential tools at your disposal. If you keep a separate journal, you'll have more space in which to record important information. If the idea of keeping a journal does not appeal to you, then think of it as keeping a progress report. I have seen successful clients use everything from day planner notations and long handwritten entries in flower-covered journals to computer spreadsheets and entries on their cell phone.

Do not underestimate the impact a journal (or progress report) will have on improving your performance. Use it to monitor your food, activities, exercise and general progress—mentally, physically, spiritually and in terms of your relationships. Use it to record and build on your successes. Remember to record what you did well. Ask yourself, "Did I change anything today?" Give yourself a high five for moving one inch closer to your goal, whether you did something constructive (example: you completed your 10 minutes of activity for the day) or you avoided doing something that would have been counterproductive (example: you skipped the triple-layer birthday cake). Also, be sure to write down your feelings. They may reveal more than you expect—if not immediately, then over time.

Not long ago, one of my son's baseball coaches told me about a secret he learned when interviewing some of the very best players in the major leagues. He found that these players rarely, if ever, watched footage of their mistakes. Instead, they learned to watch and rewatch what they did well. This was to reinforce

Reward Yourself

Positive reinforcement is a wonderful thing. It works for puppies, it works for people—and it will work for you even if you're the one supplying your own pat on the back. At the end of each week, after you've earned a certain number of check marks, treat yourself to something that does not have a lot of calories. What would you most enjoy?

- A movie in
- A movie out
- A manicure
- A fruit smoothie
- Fancy soap
- Fresh spices
- New candles
- A massage
- Time to yourself
- Time with a friend

Decide in advance when you'll let yourself go on a shopping spree for new clothes to fit the new you. Some of my clients are really delighted to go shopping for their new body as soon as possible, while others wait until they reach their goal weight.

mentally what they needed to do to be successful. I thought: What a great concept! Focus on the positive and forget about the negative. Of course! Maybe this simple strategy will help encourage my clients to track their progress. So I began to ask my clients to track what they did well, write it down and repeat it over and over again. And you know what? It helped—a lot.

To get you started on your own tracking system, I suggest that you check off each activity in the daily instructions right on the pages in Chapter 10. You could use check marks, plus or minus signs, or even smiley faces. The benefit of checking off your workouts is that, as time passes and the check marks add up, you'll have a visible reminder of all your previous successes.

Find Support

Here's a trivia question for you: What do Bill Gates, Tiger Woods and Oprah Winfrey have in common? It's not just "success." It's that they all attribute their personal success to a mentor or coach, someone who instructed, encouraged, pushed, trained and otherwise brought out the best in them. Similarly, when it comes to attaining our personal health and fitness goals, researchers have found that coaching, ongoing support and accountability are crucial to sustaining progress.

As I mentioned earlier, you'll want to find partners to walk beside you during this journey. Choose a person, or people, with whom you can share your highs and lows. Let your friends know that you're going to need their support. Talk to your mom every Sunday, ask her how she is and then tell her how you're doing. Ask your brother or sister to hold you accountable. Enlist your kids in your daily workout routine.

Friends, loved ones or coaches can encourage you and keep you honest, so "buddy up" with someone as you transform yourself. Because working with other people can be so helpful, I've included a separate section on how to put together a health and fitness group (see Chapter 11).

Don't Give Up

To tell you the truth, it's very rare for someone to drop out of my 4•3•2•1 program. The 10-minute workouts are manageable for everyone. Once you get started, you'll feel so much better that you won't want to stop. But if you follow the numbers on your bathroom scale, it's natural to occasionally hit a plateau. If this happens to you, stay on the program—and toss the scale! Your body can continue to change and improve even if your weight stays the same. Are your clothes fitting better? Do you have more energy? The scale is only one way to measure your success—and not a very good one, at that.

If you slip up one day and eat too much of the wrong thing, or miss a workout, don't let it get you down. What a waste it would be to throw away your efforts so far. Beating yourself up over the occasional lapse will accomplish nothing. Just wake up the next morning and welcome the opportunity to get back on track. Nobody's perfect.

Your 4·3·2·1 Starting Point

There is no specific body type, physique or athletic accomplishment that defines fitness. "Being fit" means having the strength and vitality you need to perform your daily activities—going to work, running your business, taking care of your children, enjoying your favorite hobbies—without undue fatigue. It means having the energy to pursue your life goals. It is a state of being that helps you live life to its fullest.

Your current level of fitness will have an effect on the way you use this book. I'm expecting that the vast majority of readers will begin the 10-Minute Total Body Breakthrough program right at the beginning: Level I. There are many reasons why this is a good idea:

- I have carefully constructed the 4·3·2·1 workouts so they get more challenging as you progress through all three levels of the program.

- Each level has 28 days of instructions. The different activities you are asked to do each day have a cumulative effect. If you start in the middle, you will miss out.

- Similarly, all of the tips at every level—how to use food as fuel for your body, how to manage stress, how to get the support you need, and so on—will contribute to your long-term success.

- When you begin at the beginning, you have 12 weeks in which to make your 4·3·2·1 workouts a new habit. By the end of the program, you will enjoy your fitness regimen and it will fit seamlessly into your life.

- Don't forget the benefit of tracking your progress and experiences for a full 12 weeks. The longer you pay attention to the strategies that work for you, the more successful you will be.

In general, you should start at Level I if:

- It's been at least two months since you've exercised with any regularity.

- You currently do push-ups and sit-ups every day but don't do any cardiovascular exercise, resistance training, core-strengthening exercises or stretching.

- You currently do 30 minutes of cardiovascular activity (walking, running, elliptical machine, stair climbing, rowing) three days per week but perform a minimal amount of resistance training, core-strengthening exercises or stretching.

On the other hand, if you have been working out for years and cardiovascular exercise, lifting weights, core-strengthening exercises and stretching are a regular part of your life, you can start at Level II or even at Level III. But be sure to complete the fitness and overall health assessments included in this chapter before deciding to skip a level or before starting a new one.

In the pages that follow, you will determine exactly how fit you are and learn how to adapt the 4·3·2·1 program to your fitness level and personal preferences.

Reasons to Consult Your Physician

Almost everyone can safely do some form of exercise. However, you should consult your doctor before beginning this program if you're pregnant or if you have any health issues, such as high blood pressure, heart trouble, chest pain, dizzy spells or a serious bone or joint problem. If you are currently taking medications, work with your health care professional to adjust your dosages as you become healthier.

4·3·2·1 FITNESS ASSESSMENT

Your answers to the questions in the chart below will help you determine your current fitness level. In some cases, you may need to consult the fitness tests on pages 80 through 84.

Each "yes" answer to the questions in the chart is worth 10 points. Add up your score to assess your fitness level and see how you should proceed with the 4•3•2•1 program.

Your Current Fitness Level

1. Do you perform cardiovascular exercises, such as walking, cycling, jogging, swimming or jumping rope, at least four times a week?
☐ Yes ☐ No

2. Would you rate your cardiovascular endurance as good to excellent? (*Optional: To determine your score, perform the One-Mile Endurance Walk on page 80.*)
☐ Yes ☐ No

3. Do you perform resistance training exercises, such as push-ups or routines using free weights, dumbbells or resistance bands, at least two times a week?
☐ Yes ☐ No

4. Would you rate your current upper-body strength as good to excellent? (*Optional: To determine your score, perform the Push-Up Test on pages 80–81.*)
☐ Yes ☐ No

5. Do you perform core exercises to strengthen your abdominal and lower back muscles, such as sit-ups or crunches, at least four times a week?
☐ Yes ☐ No

6. Would you rate your abdominal strength as good to excellent? (*Optional: To determine your score, perform the Partial Curl-Up Test on pages 81–82.*)
☐ Yes ☐ No

7. Do you regularly perform stretching exercises for the upper and lower body, such as overhead arm stretches, hamstring, calf or quadriceps stretches, at least four times a week?
☐ Yes ☐ No

8. Would you rate your flexibility as good to excellent? (*Optional: To determine your score, perform the Sit-and-Reach Flexibility Test on pages 82–83.*)
☐ Yes ☐ No

9. Would you rate your current BMI (see page 83) as good to excellent? (*To determine your BMI, see page 83.*)
☐ Yes ☐ No

10. Would you rate your overall fitness level as good to excellent? (*See page 84 for the results of any tests you took to determine your current fitness level.*)
☐ Yes ☐ No

Your Score	Where You Should Begin	Recommendations
0 to 50	Level I	Follow the daily instructions for Level I. Perform one 4•3•2•1 workout every other day. On alternate days, do 10 minutes of cardiovascular exercise or another physical activity that you enjoy.
51 to 70	Level I	Follow the daily instructions for Level I. Perform one to three sets of a Level I workout every other day, using the tips that make the exercises more challenging. If you already have a cardiovascular fitness regimen, follow it on alternate days.
71 to 90	Level II	Read the daily instructions for Level I, then skip to Level II. Perform one to three sets of a Level II workout every other day. If you wish, use the tips that make the exercises more challenging. If you already have a cardiovascular fitness regimen, follow it on alternate days.
91 to 100	Level III	Read the daily instructions for Levels I and II, then skip to Level III. Perform one to four sets of a Level III workout every other day. If you wish, use the tips that make the exercises more challenging. If you already have a cardiovascular fitness regimen, follow it on alternate days.

The Fitness Tests

If you choose to do the tests on the pages that follow, you will be able to quantify your current fitness in terms of aerobic capacity, upper body and abdominal strength and endurance, and flexibility. In the future, you'll have a baseline for comparison. If your results are discouraging now, this means there's lots of room for improvement—and you'll feel that much better the next time you evaluate your fitness.

These assessments will also provide a motivational tool. They will help you:

- Identify your strengths and weaknesses.

- Determine your personal goals.

- Monitor your progress throughout the program.

- Know when you're ready to increase your level of intensity.

One-Mile Endurance Walk

This test will evaluate your aerobic capacity—that is, it will determine the strength of your heart by measuring its efficiency in delivering oxygen to working muscles.

Equipment Needed: Sneakers and a watch with a second hand or a stopwatch or timer

Goal: To complete a one-mile walk in the fastest time possible

Instructions:

- Find a track or safe area that can be accurately marked for one mile.

- Warm up for approximately 5 to 10 minutes by performing light walking.

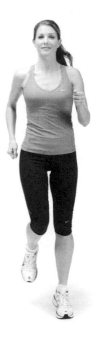

- After completing your warm-up, start your timer and begin the endurance walk.

- Move as fast as you can, at a walk, for one mile. No running!

- If you experience any pain, severe shortness of breath or abnormal signs, stop.

- At the end of the one-mile distance, note your finish time to the closest second.

Results:

If you completed your walk in 16 minutes or more, you currently have *low* cardiovascular fitness.

If you completed your walk in 13 to 15 minutes, you currently have *average* cardiovascular fitness.

If you completed your walk in 12 minutes or less, you currently have *good/excellent* cardiovascular fitness.

Push-Up Test

This test will determine the strength and endurance of your upper-body muscles. Do not attempt this assessment if you have shoulder pain, lower back pain or uncontrolled high blood pressure.

Equipment Needed: Exercise mat (optional)

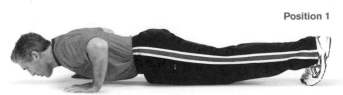

Position 1

Goal: To complete as many push-ups as possible without rest

Instructions:

■ To get the most out of this test, warm up your shoulders before you start the exercise. Begin by performing a light aerobic movement such as walking or marching in place (to raise your body temperature) for 3 to 5 minutes. Next, perform a combination of shoulder movements to increase blood flow and increase joint mobility: 1) *Forward shoulder rolls.* Shrug your shoulders up toward your ears and make forward circular motions with your shoulders. 2) *Backward shoulder rolls.* Shrug your shoulders up toward your ears and make backward circular motions with your shoulders. 3) *Arm rotations.* Move your hands and arms in a circular motion in front of your body or reaching behind your body.

■ Lie on your stomach with your legs together and your back straight. Position your hands, pointing forward, under your shoulders. (**Position 1**)

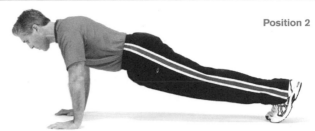

Position 2

■ Push up your body by straightening your arms, keeping your back and body straight. (**Position 2**) Men place their weight on their hands and toes, while women place their weight on their hands and knees.

■ Return to your starting position, but let only your chin touch the floor (your chest, hips and legs should not touch the floor).

■ Perform as many consecutive push-ups as you can without undue strain and without stopping to rest. Count how many times your chin touches the floor.

■ There is no time limit. Stop the test if you feel excessive strain or are unable to maintain proper form.

Norms for Push-Up Test Results

For men

Age	20–29	30–39	40–49	50–59	60–69
Excellent	36+	30+	25+	21+	18+
Very good	35–29	29–22	24–17	20–13	17–11
Good	28–22	21–17	16–13	12–10	10–8
Fair	21–17	16–12	12–10	9–7	7–5
Needs improvement	<16	<11	<9	<6	<4

For women

Age	20–29	30–39	40–49	50–59	60–69
Excellent	30+	27+	24+	21+	17+
Very good	29–21	26–20	23–15	20–11	16–12
Good	20–15	19–13	14–11	10–7	11–5
Fair	14–10	12–8	10–5	6–2	4–2
Needs improvement	<9	<7	<4	<1	<1

Partial Curl-Up Test

You'll need a partner for this test, which will determine the muscular strength/endurance of your abdominal muscles.

Equipment Needed: Cushioned surface or mat (optional); ruler; masking tape; watch with a second hand or a stopwatch or timer.

Goal: To complete as many partial (one-quarter) curl-ups as possible in 1 minute.

Instructions:

■ Begin by performing a light aerobic movement such as walking or marching in place (in order to raise your body temperature) for 3 to 5 minutes. Next, to prepare your abdominal muscles and your lower back for this test, lie down on your back and perform 8 to 10 slow abdominal crunches (see page 108).

■ Lie on your back with your arms fully extended along your sides, palms down. Lift your head and touch your chin. Have a partner mark the floor with masking tape at the ends of your fingertips. Measure 3 inches beyond this mark and place an object—a block of wood, for example, or a book—as a touch reference point. (**Position 1**)

■ With your knees bent and your feet shoulder-width apart, press the small of your back to the floor, tighten your abdominal muscles and lift your head and shoulders without letting the small of your back leave the floor. As you raise your head and shoulders, your hands must slide at least 3 inches forward to your touch point to qualify for a successful curl-up. Be careful not to slide your body forward (shortening the distance to your touch point). (**Position 2**) Return your shoulders to the mat before starting another curl-up.

■ Count the number of consecutive partial curl-ups you can do in 1 minute, without undue strain and without stopping to rest.

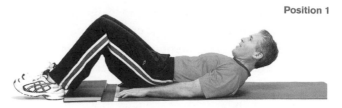

Position 1

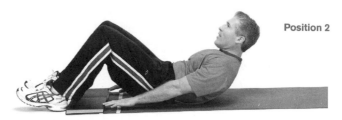

Position 2

Norms for Partial Curl-Up Test

For men

Age	15–19	20–29	30–39	40–49	50–59	60+
Excellent	60+	54+	45+	39+	33+	29+
Good	53	46	39	33	28	21
Average	48	41	34	28	23	15
Fair	41	36	28	21	16	9
Poor	<41	<36	<28	<21	<16	<9

For women

Age	15–19	20–29	30–39	40–49	50–59	60+
Excellent	53+	45+	36+	31+	24+	20+
Good	45	39	30	25	15	15
Average	40	31	25	19	6	5
Fair	34	26	19	9	4	2
Poor	<34	<26	<19	<9	<4	<2

Sit-and-Reach Flexibility Test

This test will determine the flexibility of your lower back and leg muscles.

Equipment Needed: Yardstick or measuring tape; masking tape

Goal: To bend forward as far as you can while sitting on the floor with your legs in front of you

Instructions:

■ Select a surface that is flat and comfortable.

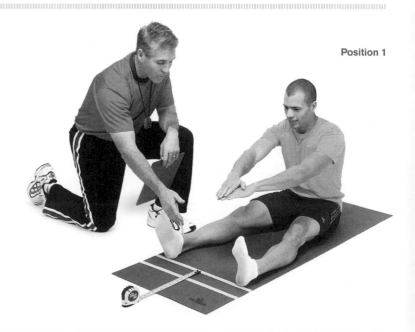

Position 1

- Mark a line on the floor using at least 12 inches of masking tape. Then mark an additional line 3 inches beyond the first one.

- Place one hand on top of the other, both palms facing down. (**Position 1**) Exhale and reach toward the second line or past it while keeping your legs straight. (**Position 2**)

- Perform this test four times, recording the fourth attempt.

- Measure, in inches, the distance you reach past the second line as "+" or before the line as "–".

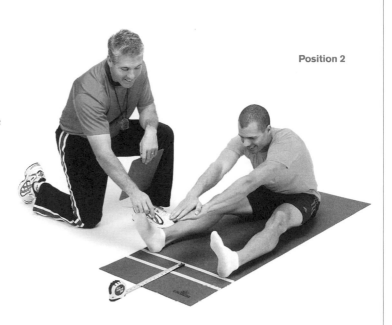

Position 2

Results:

If you can reach 3 or more inches past the second line, consider yourself in the good-to-excellent category for flexibility.

What Is Your BMI?

BMI stands for Body Mass Index, a measurement of your total body fat. This measurement is used to screen weight categories that may lead to health problems. The higher your BMI, the more worried about your health you should be. For most people, the BMI offers a better picture of overall health and fitness than numbers on the bathroom scale. (For athletes and individuals who are very muscular, the results from the BMI chart can be misleading, because the weight of their muscle tissue can place them in a higher category.)

- A healthy BMI for adults is between 18.5 and 25.

- A BMI higher than 25 is considered overweight.

- A BMI over 30 is considered obese.

  To find your BMI:

- *Determine your height.* Have a friend or family member measure you without shoes on. Standing on tiptoe is not allowed. Stand tall with your eyes looking straight ahead.

- *Determine your weight.* Weigh yourself first thing in the morning, preferably without clothes on. Place the scale on a flat, hard surface. If possible, use the same scale throughout your 10-Minute Total Body Breakthrough program—but don't look at it often. I promise you will lose fat and gain muscle on a steady, consistent basis by following the daily instructions.

- *Determine your BMI category* (healthy weight, overweight or obese). In the chart on the next page, you'll see that the loss of 5 or 10 pounds can take you from the overweight category to the healthy weight category. For example, if you are 5'9" tall and weigh 175 pounds, you are overweight: If you lose 10 pounds, your weight will be in the healthy range.

The Body Mass Index

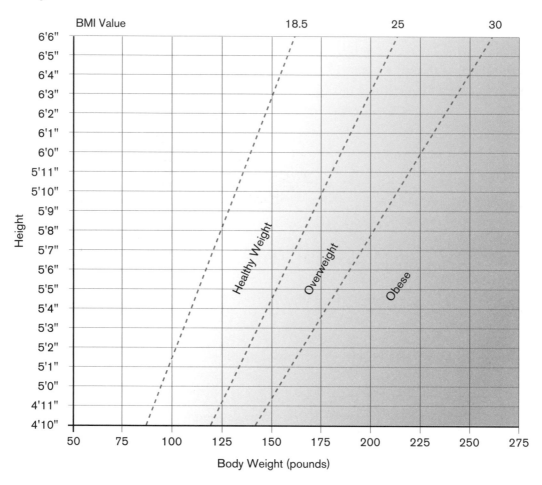

Your Fitness Test Results

Any reputable fitness program must include assessment. Record the results of your fitness tests below. After completing Level I (and Levels II and III), perform the tests again and record your improved results. This will provide you with incontrovertible evidence that all your efforts are yielding wonderful results.

One-Mile Endurance Walk
I successfully completed my one-mile endurance walk in _____ minutes.

Push-Up Test
I successfully completed _____ push-ups.

Partial Curl-Up Test
I successfully completed _____ partial curl-ups in 1 minute.

Sit-and-Reach Flexibility Test
I was able to reach _____ inches
    □ before
    □ beyond
the tape on the floor.

Body Mass Index (BMI)
My height is _____.
My weight is _____.
My BMI category is _____.

YOUR CURRENT HEALTH STATUS

Congratulations, you just completed the "fitness portion" of this assessment! Now let's take a snapshot of your overall health.

In this next section, you'll have the opportunity to complete a number of tests that will provide an excellent barometer of how healthy you are right now. Used as regular follow-up tests, these "success markers" will show you how your 10-Minute Total Body Breakthrough is making significant improvements in every area of your life. First measure your waist and hips. Next take your blood pressure. After that, you'll have the option of getting your cholesterol, glucose and triglycerides checked, as well as some additional suggested health tests. Last, I encourage you to take "before" and "after" photos of yourself and sign the commitment form on page 88. (Don't worry, you'll be promising nothing more than to move your body 10 minutes a day and to use food as fuel.)

Determine Your Waist/Hip Ratio

Over time, most of us accumulate excess fat around the waist and hips, and where this excess body fat is stored has significant implications. The higher your waist/hip ratio, the greater your risk for hypertension, heart disease and type 2 diabetes. Measuring your waist/hip ratio also gives you a handy way of monitoring your progress as you become more fit.

To accurately determine your waist/hip ratio:

■ *Measure your waist.* Stand with your feet together. Hold your arms out at shoulder level. Have a friend place a measuring tape lightly but firmly around your waist, positioned at your naval, parallel to the floor. Exhale—because your belly expands when you breathe in—and record your waist measurement, to the nearest quarter of an inch, in the space below.

■ *Measure your hips.* Now have your friend place the measuring tape around the widest point

of your hips (that is, around the widest part of your butt). Record your hip measurement, to the nearest quarter of an inch, in the space below.

■ *Divide your waist measurement by your hip measurement.* (If you don't have a calculator handy, visit the Waist/Hip Ratio Calculator at www.4321fitness.com.) Record your waist/hip ratio in the space below.

My waist measurement is _____ inches.
My hip measurement is _____ inches.
My waist/hip ratio is _____.

Women: If your waist/hip ratio is greater than 0.8, you are at increased risk for heart disease, diabetes, high blood pressure and stroke.

Men: If your waist/hip ratio is greater than 1.0, you are at increased risk for heart disease, diabetes, high blood pressure and stroke.

Determine Your Blood Pressure

Blood pressure represents the force that your blood exerts upon the walls of your blood vessels, especially your arteries. High blood pressure, which can be caused by the buildup of plaque on artery walls, makes the heart work harder and over time increases the risk of stroke, heart attack, heart failure, an arterial aneurysm or kidney failure. Even moderately elevated blood pressure will shorten your life expectancy. Extremely high blood pressure, if left untreated, is fatal within a few years, especially when combined with smoking, obesity, high cholesterol or diabetes. High blood pressure is often referred to as a "silent killer" because it typically has no obvious symptoms.

Usually a health professional puts a blood pressure cuff on your arm, inflates the cuff to restrict the flow of blood, then loosens the cuff, and listens to your blood with a stethoscope as it resumes flowing

---

Take a "Before" Photo

Nothing is more motivating than viewing the changes in your appearance that will occur over the next 12 weeks. Ask a friend or family member to take "before" and "after" pictures for you. To create the most effective photos:

- Don't stand too close to the camera. You want a picture of your entire body.

- Don't stand too far from the camera— your image will be too small.

- Wear clothing that shows your physique clearly, such as a swimsuit or gym shorts with a fitted T-shirt or tank top.

- Have a blank surface behind you, such as a white wall or sheet.

- Take both your "before" and "after" photos in the same location.

We want to show you off! If you like, you can upload your "before" and "after" pictures at www.4321fitness.com, and we'll try to share your story and pictures to help motivate others with your amazing changes.

---

normally. There are also electronic machines that will take a blood pressure reading from a cuff that inflates on your arm. Some pharmacies have do-it-yourself blood pressure monitors, and you also can purchase a blood pressure monitor for home use. Not all monitors are equally accurate.

Blood pressure results can vary according to the method used to obtain them. Also, if the cuff is too small or too large, the results will be inaccurate. It's important to know that your results can vary from one arm to the other. They can also depend on your state of mind; if the doctor's office makes you very nervous, you may get a so-called "white coat" blood pressure reading that is artificially elevated because of your situational distress.

Blood pressure is given as two figures: systolic and diastolic. The reading on the gauge when blood flow is first heard is called the *systolic* pressure; this represents the peak blood pressure that occurs when your heart contracts. The reading on the gauge when blood flow can no longer be heard

is the *diastolic* pressure; this represents the lower blood pressure that occurs when the heart relaxes between beats. If your systolic pressure is 120 mm Hg and your diastolic pressure is 80 mm Hg, your blood pressure is recorded as 120/80 and described as "120 over 80."

Systolic	Diastolic	Risk Classification
Below 120	Below 80	Normal
120 to 139	80 to 89	Prehypertension
140 to 159	90 to 99	Stage 1 hypertension
Above 160	Above 100	Stage 2 hypertension

The American Heart Association estimates that high blood pressure affects approximately one in three adults in the United States—73 million people. What causes high blood pressure is not entirely clear. Some people have a genetic predisposition for hypertension, while in other people it's associated with poor eating habits, excess dietary salt, obesity or a sedentary lifestyle. Making dietary changes and getting more exercise can successfully reduce high blood pressure, even if you have a genetic link to this disease.

My systolic blood pressure is _____.

My diastolic blood pressure is _____.

My blood pressure is:

☐ Normal

☐ Somewhat high—medication is not yet necessary

☐ Too high—I am on medication

Baseline Bloodwork: Glucose, Cholesterol and Triglycerides

We often do a comprehensive bloodwork analysis on our fitness clients, using 40 different parameters. If you're interested in obtaining a complete analysis of your blood, consult your doctor or go to a health and fitness facility that offers bloodwork. Unless you are a health professional, you will need someone to interpret the detailed results for you.

At a minimum, I recommend obtaining the following information about your blood chemistry for the 10-Minute Total Body Breakthrough program. Record your results in the space provided.

- **Your fasting blood glucose level.** A normal result is between 70 and 99 mg/dl.

- **Your total cholesterol.** You can interpret your results as follows:

Total Cholesterol	Risk Classification
Below 200 mg/dl	Desirable
200 to 239 mg/dl	Borderline
240 mg/dl and above	Undesirable

- **Your high-density lipoprotein (HDL) or "good" cholesterol.** HDL cholesterol transports "bad" cholesterol from the blood to the liver, where it is excreted by the body. The higher the number, the better, since HDL has a protective role in guarding against heart disease.

Total HDL ("Good") Cholesterol	Risk Classification
60 mg/dl and above	Desirable
40 to 60 mg/dl	Acceptable
Below 40 mg/dl	Undesirable

- **Your low-density lipoprotein (LDL) or "bad" cholesterol.** LDL cholesterol tends to linger in the blood and can build up on the walls of your arteries, increasing your chances of heart attack and stroke. The lower your number, the better.

Total LDL ("Bad") Cholesterol	Risk Classification
Below 100 mg/dl	Desirable
100 to 129 mg/dl	Acceptable
130 to 159 mg/dl	Borderline
160 to 189 mg/dl	Undesirable
190 mg/dl or above	Very undesirable

Your cholesterol results may be given as a ratio of your total cholesterol to your HDL cholesterol. This ratio is obtained by dividing the HDL cholesterol level into the total cholesterol. For example, if a person's total cholesterol is 200 mg/dl, with an HDL cholesterol level of 50 mg/dl, the ratio would be

4:1. A healthy ratio is below 5:1; the optimum ratio is 3.5:1. It's also possible to obtain the ratio of your LDL cholesterol to your HDL cholesterol. In this case, the ratio should be below 3.5. Please note that the American Heart Association recommends using absolute numbers for cholesterol, rather than ratios. Absolute numbers give doctors a better idea of what type of treatment is needed by the patient.

- **Your serum triglycerides.** High levels of the circulating fats called triglycerides are also a risk factor for heart disease. You can interpret your results as follows:

Triglycerides	Risk Classification
Below 150 mg/dl	Desirable
150 to 199 mg/dl	Borderline
200 to 499 mg/dl	Undesirable
500 or above	Very undesirable

Your Bloodwork Results

Write your baseline results for your first bloodwork below. The next time you have your blood analyzed, you'll be happy to see the results improve.

My fasting blood glucose level is _____.

My total cholesterol is _____.

My HDL ("good") cholesterol is _____.

My LDL ("bad") cholesterol is _____.

My serum triglycerides are _____.

Additional Health Assessments

Assembling the total picture of your health is like putting together an image using different numbers of pixels. The pixels are your test results. You can get a general, somewhat fuzzy picture of your health using a few large pixels. Adding more pixels will yield a more focused picture. If you really want to closely analyze the picture of your health, you need an image made up of dozens of pixels.

Your doctor, health professional or fitness center will be able to give you additional tests that will help you complete the total picture of your current health and fitness. These include:

- Additional cardiovascular endurance tests

- Additional muscular strength tests

- Lung function test

- Your resting heart rate

- Your bone density

Are You Ready to Make a Commitment?

Please fill out the commitment pledge to yourself below. Remember to add your starting date. As the weeks go by and you become more fit, this date will become more important to you.

You may want to post a copy of this document on your refrigerator or keep it in your wallet. Written contracts are powerful—even the ones you make with yourself.

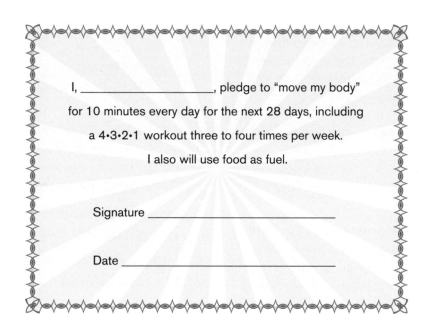

I, _____, pledge to "move my body"

for 10 minutes every day for the next 28 days, including

a 4•3•2•1 workout three to four times per week.

I also will use food as fuel.

Signature _____

Date _____

chapter 7

Level I: Now You're Moving!

Fitness Using Bodyweight

This is it! You're ready to begin. In the pages that follow, you'll find your first four 10-minute workouts. Each workout consists of 4 minutes of H.E.A.T., 3 minutes of resistance exercise, 2 minutes of core-strengthening exercises and 1 minute of stretching and deep breathing. Every exercise has written instructions, "how-to" photographs, guidelines for maintaining perfect form and tips to make the exercise either easier or harder, depending on your level of fitness.

Level I is devoted to exercises that are done using bodyweight—no equipment required. This means you can perform the workouts in this chapter whenever and wherever you like, indoors or out. Once you become familiar with all the different exercises, you may find yourself doing some easy stretches while waiting at the airport, a few abdominal crunches while watching television, or a couple of lunges at work after a long meeting leaves you bored stiff—literally!

Use a Mat for Extra Comfort

All the exercises in Level I are based on bodyweight, so no exercise equipment is required, but you may want to invest in an exercise mat for extra protection and comfort. Today you can choose from Pilates, aerobic and/or yoga mats for floor exercises. Pilates mats provide the most cushioning. The thinner yoga mats are sticky, to prevent slipping. I recommend an exercise mat that measures at least half an inch and up to two inches in thickness. Make sure the mat is large enough for your body in length and width. Most exercise mats can be purchased for under $30. Go to your local sporting goods store or visit my website, www.4321fitness.com, and select from one of our trustworthy partner fitness equipment stores. Or, if your floor is carpeted, you can just lay down a towel instead.

Keep Time During Your Workouts

As you understand by now, each of the four sections of the 10-Minute Total Body Breakthrough workout involves specific times:

- When you're doing your 4 minutes of H.E.A.T., you alternate 30 seconds of intense activity with 30 seconds of moderate activity. You need a way to know when 30 seconds have passed and it's time to switch.

- In the resistance and core-strengthening sections, each exercise lasts 1 minute. You need to know when to stop one exercise and quickly move on to the next.

- The stretching and deep breathing section is broken down into two 30-second exercises, so again you need a way to know when to switch.

My clients have been extremely resourceful when it comes to using different timing methods. Try one of the following approaches until you find one that works best for you.

Large wall clock with second hand. Find an inexpensive clock—make sure it's nice and big—and mount it on a wall or place it on the floor near you. The second hand of the clock becomes the interval timer for your H.E.A.T. sessions and the rest of your 4•3•2•1 workout.

Wristwatch with second hand. Use an analog wristwatch the same way you would a wall clock.

Digital sports watch. Wristwatches of this kind allow you to start and stop different aspects of your workout with the touch of a button. Some have extra features, such as a heart rate monitor.

Stopwatch. Wear a standard stopwatch around your neck. Most stopwatches have split timers that allow you to track your total minutes for the workout as well as your intervals.

Cell phone. Most cell phones have a stopwatch feature. If you can find it in your phone's assortment of tools, you're all set.

Record your own voice. One of the most innovative ways to monitor your workouts is to use a recording device (cell phone, recorder, desktop computer or laptop computer) and a stopwatch. Record your own instructions to yourself on when to start and stop your exercising. You can even add motivational encouragement: "Okay, Sean, here we go . . . let's have a great workout today!" When a certain portion of the workout is nearly over, say: "You have 4 seconds . . . 3 seconds . . . 2 seconds . . . and *stop*. Way to go! Now move on to your next exercise." You don't even have to look at a clock—all you have to do is listen to your own voice and instructions.

Move to the Music

Nothing makes exercising more fun than adding music in the background. Crank up the volume and work it out to some of your favorites. Before you know it, you'll feel like a kid again.

How to Gauge the Level of Your Exertion During H.E.A.T.

Below is an intensity scale to help explain what level of exertion is appropriate for you to use during your sessions of H.E.A.T.

Intensity Scale

1. Easy
2. Easy/slow
3. Slow
> Very light breathing; minimal effort

4. Slow/moderate
5. Moderate
> More breathing and less conversation, like catching up to someone

6. Moderate/fast
7. Fast
8. Fast/intense
> Labored breathing, like chasing after a child or cab

9. Intense
10. High effort
> Blast off! Moving as hard and fast as you can; racing

Your H.E.A.T. cardiovascular workout will look like this:

30 seconds of moderate activity ➤ (Warm-up: Levels 1 to 3)

30 seconds of H.E.A.T. ➤ (Levels 4 to 5)

30 seconds of moderate activity ➤ (Level 3)

30 seconds of H.E.A.T. ➤ (Levels 6 to 7)

30 seconds of moderate activity ➤ (Level 4)

30 seconds of H.E.A.T. ➤ (Levels 7 to 8)

30 seconds of moderate activity ➤ (Level 5)

Final 30 seconds of H.E.A.T. ➤ (Levels 9 to 10)

Grand total: **❹ minutes** of activity

MP3 recording. If you're technologically inclined, you can record your own workout with music and your own voice on a CD or MP3 player and take it wherever you go to exercise.

Warm Up for Your Workouts

During your sessions of H.E.A.T., you will alternate faster-paced periods of activity with more moderately paced periods of activity. Ideally, you'll take 2 to 5 minutes to warm up your muscles before each workout. A proper warm-up prepares you by increasing the flow of blood (and oxygen) to your muscles, raising your body temperature, preparing your muscles to contract efficiently, decreasing muscle stiffness, increasing your range of motion and minimizing your risk of injury. Warming up also prepares you mentally by clearing your mind of day-to-day concerns and increasing your focus on the workout ahead.

To warm up your body properly, first perform a few minutes of light aerobic activity such as walking or marching in place at a moderate pace to increase your body temperature. Next, perform dynamic movements such as Jumping Jacks (page 113), Walking Lunges (page 127) or Airplanes (page 181) to most effectively prepare the muscles you will be using during your 4•3•2•1 session. Experiment and see what works best for you.

If you don't have time to warm up, you'll need to begin your H.E.A.T. sessions at a gentler pace, incorporating your warm-up into your 10-minute workout. Use the first 2 minutes of your H.E.A.T. sessions to properly warm up your body and prepare your mind.

WORKOUT 1

Welcome to 4•3•2•1 Workout 1—your first step to getting fit! This 10-minute, full-body workout is great for those who are getting back into shape. It's also good for those who have an injury or are recovering from an illness. This is a no-sweat workout (okay, some of you may "glow" a little) that you can perform at home, in your office, outdoors, in a hotel room or even when you're sitting alone in a waiting room. All the movements use just your bodyweight, so you don't need any special gym equipment. Completing one full circuit of this workout will work every major muscle group in your body *and* boost your metabolism for hours.

4 minutes | High-Energy Aerobic Training

Chair Jogging

EQUIPMENT: **Sturdy chair**
MUSCLES WORKED: **Heart, shoulders, arms, core and legs**

For today's H.E.A.T. workout, you don't even have to stand up! Chair Jogging is a great aerobic exercise that provides you with the benefits of jogging without the wear and tear on your feet, hips or knee joints.

▶ GET STARTED

Sit upright at the edge of a sturdy chair with your feet placed hip-width apart. Bend your arms at a 90° angle. (**Position 1**)

▶ GET MOVING

1. Tighten your abdominal muscles, and begin to gently move your arms and legs as if you were doing a slow jog. Your left arm and right leg go up at the same time, and vice versa. Push off from the balls of your feet— not your heels—and raise your knees as high as you comfortably can. Maintain a leisurely pace for 30 seconds. (**Position 2**)

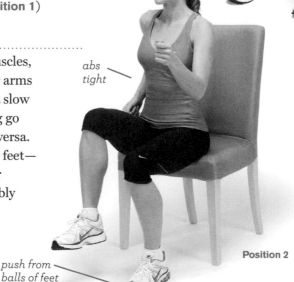

shoulders relaxed

chest up

Position 1

eyes straight ahead

abs tight

push from balls of feet

Position 2

2. Now, bending forward slightly from the waist, perform the same motion, but faster. Move your arms and legs as rapidly as you comfortably can. Maintain a brisk pace for 30 seconds. (**Position 3**)

3. Keep alternating, slow and fast, every 30 seconds for a total of 4 minutes. Try to make your "slow" periods progressively a little faster and your "fast" periods even faster. For the last 30 seconds, challenge yourself!

Too hard? Tone it down
• Keep your hands on your hips throughout the movement.
• Move more slowly.

Too easy? Kick it up
• Move your arms and legs more quickly during both the slow and fast portions of the exercise.
• Hold water bottles or other weighted objects in your hands as you "jog."

TAKE 10 TIPS

Even a simple move should be done using the proper form. And don't forget to breathe. Holding your breath will not make the 4 minutes go faster!

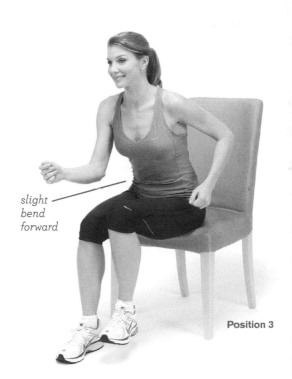

slight bend forward

Position 3

❸ minutes | Resistance Exercise

Stationary Wall Squat

EQUIPMENT: **Wall or other fixed object**
MUSCLES WORKED: **Legs, butt and core**

This is an exercise that can be done wherever there's a wall—in your office during a conference call, in your kitchen when you're cooking dinner, in your bathroom while the kids are finishing up in the tub or while waiting in line at a movie theater.

▶ GET STARTED

Lean against a smooth wall with your feet hip-width apart and your arms at your sides. Walk your feet out from the wall 2 to 3 feet in front of you and bend your knees slightly. (**Position 1**)

▶ GET MOVING

1. Keeping your chest up and your back against the wall, bend both knees and slide down as low as you comfortably can.

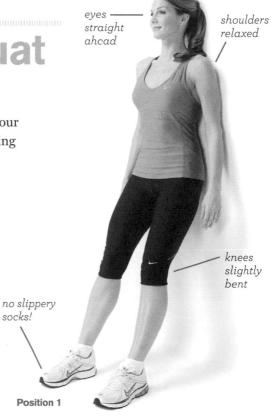

eyes straight ahead
shoulders relaxed
knees slightly bent
no slippery socks!

Position 1

2. When you reach the squat position, do not let your knees extend over your toes. You should be able to draw an imaginary vertical line from the top of your knees down through the middle of your feet. If necessary, move your feet farther away from the wall and start over. (**Position 2**)

3. Try to hold the wall squat for 1 minute.

Too hard? Tone it down

- Don't go so far into the squat. You can start with a quarter-squat. In time, you'll be able to go lower.
- Keep your hands on your hips.
- Hold the pose for less than 1 minute.
- Take a rest and then perform the wall squat again.

Too easy? Kick it up

- Go lower into your squat.
- Place your arms over your head. Imagine you're making a "touchdown" signal with both arms straight up. Your thumbs should be pointed toward the wall and your palms facing each other. Keep your shoulders down.
- Hold a single weighted object, such as a purse, a briefcase or a frying pan, with both hands overhead.

- Hold two weighted objects, such as water bottles or paperweights, one in each hand overhead.
- Once you're in the squat, slowly raise your left knee toward your waist, bringing your left foot a few inches off the ground. Transfer your body weight to your right foot. To increase the challenge, raise your left knee even higher. Try to hold this position for 30 seconds, then switch legs and hold for another 30 seconds.
- Hold the squat for more than 1 minute.

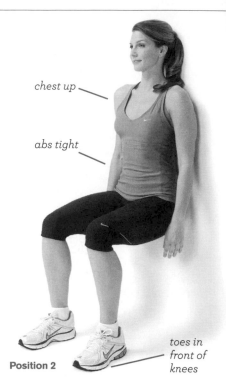

chest up

abs tight

toes in front of knees

Position 2

TAKE 10 TIPS

Be careful about your form; otherwise, you can put unnecessary pressure on your knees and other parts of your body. Remember to breathe comfortably throughout the exercise.

Wall Push-Up

EQUIPMENT: **Wall or other fixed object**
MUSCLES WORKED: **Chest, shoulders, arms and core**

Like the Stationary Wall Squat, the Wall Push-Up can be done wherever there is a wall. This exercise transforms the military push-up into an easier motion. You'll get all the benefits of the classic push-up—toned and stronger arms, chest, abdominals and lower back—without getting down on the floor.

▶ GET STARTED

Place your hands against a wall in a push-up position, fingers wide, pointing up and slightly to the sides, with both hands a little wider than shoulder-width apart and at shoulder level. Next, walk both feet back 2 to 3 feet, allowing your body to lean into the wall. Your elbows should be slightly bent and your head in alignment with your upper body. This is your starting position. (**Position 1**)

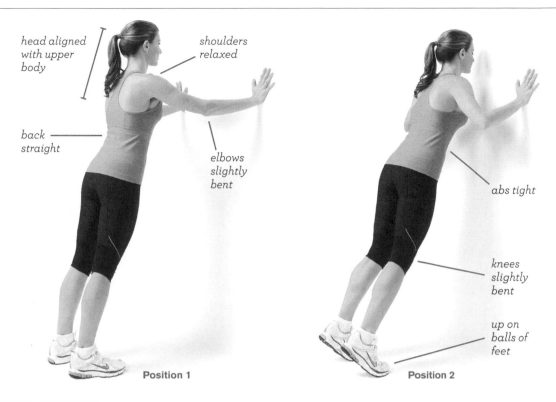

head aligned with upper body

shoulders relaxed

back straight

elbows slightly bent

abs tight

knees slightly bent

up on balls of feet

Position 1

Position 2

▶ GET MOVING

1. Rise up on the balls of your feet, leaning farther into the wall. With your knees slightly bent, lower your face and chest slowly toward the wall by bending both elbows. Imagine that your goal is to touch your forehead and nose to the wall. Go as far as you comfortably can. (**Position 2**)

2. Now extend both arms. Exhale as you press your hands into the wall and push yourself back to the starting position.

3. Perform as many Wall Push-Ups as you can in 1 minute.

> **TAKE 10 TIPS**
>
> Breathe comfortably, exhaling as you push away from the wall and straighten your arms. Proper form is important.

Too hard? Tone it down

- Go down only a quarter of the way. Remember that you don't have to touch your forehead or chest to the wall to make this exercise effective.
- Walk closer to the wall, reducing the weight on your upper body.

Too easy? Kick it up

- Move your upper body as close to the wall as you can.
- Walk both feet farther away from the wall to increase the weight on your upper body.

- Place your hands closer together on the wall. This simple adjustment increases the demand on the backs of your arms significantly, causing the triceps to work extra hard when you push back to the starting position. Good-bye "jiggle arms"!
- Do a one-armed Wall Push-Up. Place one hand behind your back and put all your weight on the hand positioned on the wall. You may want to bring your feet a little closer to the wall, as this variation is significantly more challenging. Try to perform as many one-armed push-ups as you can for 30 seconds, then switch arms for another 30 seconds.

- Do a one-legged Wall Push-Up. Raise one knee toward your chest, transferring all your weight to the other leg and tightening your abdominal muscles. Now do your Wall Push-Ups. Once you've performed as many reps as you can for 30 seconds, switch legs and perform as many as you can for 30 more seconds.
- Perform push-ups explosively, pushing up as fast as you can. This increases the total number of repetitions you complete in 1 minute and also recruits more muscle fibers in the arms, chest and shoulders.

Stationary Lunge

EQUIPMENT: Optional: chair or wall for balance
MUSCLES WORKED: Legs and butt

The lunge is my favorite lower body exercise. You can do it while you're talking on the phone, standing in line or waiting for the kids' soccer game to start. Not only does it tone and firm the entire lower body, it also helps to raise up the buttocks—when we all know they want to go south! The Stationary Lunge minimizes wear and tear of the joints and is easier for a beginner than the standard lunge. For this exercise, you get into a lunge position and hold it. The standard lunge involves repeated lowering and standing (yes, you'll get to it later).

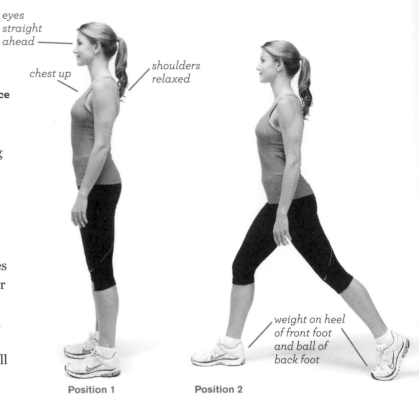

eyes straight ahead

chest up

shoulders relaxed

weight on heel of front foot and ball of back foot

Position 1   **Position 2**

▶ GET STARTED

While standing next to a chair or wall for balance or with your arms comfortably at your sides (**Position 1**), step backward 3 to 4 feet with your left foot. Press into the floor with the heel of your right foot in front and the ball of your left foot in back. With your back straight, balance your weight evenly between your front right heel and the ball of your left foot. Keep your chest up and look straight ahead. (**Position 2**)

▶ GET MOVING

1. Bend both knees, lowering your right thigh until it's parallel to the floor. Tighten your buttocks and lunge down as low as you can. Do not allow your left knee to rest on the floor. (**Position 3**) Try to hold this position for 30 seconds.

2. It's very important not to extend your right knee beyond the toes of your right foot. If this happens, try a longer stance by moving your left foot a little farther back, and reevaluate the position of your front knee. You should be able to draw an imaginary vertical line from your front knee to the middle of your front foot.

3. Next, extend both legs and push yourself back to the starting position.

4. Now lunge with the other leg. Try to hold your position for 30 seconds.

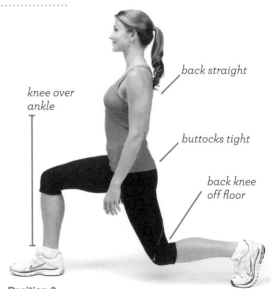

knee over ankle

back straight

buttocks tight

back knee off floor

Position 3

Too hard? Tone it down

- Don't go so far into the lunge. Instead of trying to lower your front thigh to a position parallel with the floor, begin with a quarter-lunge. Bend your front and back legs slightly.

- Keep your hands on your hips.

- Take a rest and then perform the lunge again.

Too easy? Kick it up

- Go lower in your lunge.

- Place your arms over your head. Imagine you're making a "touchdown" signal with both arms straight up. Pull your shoulder blades together, but keep your shoulders down. This motion increases the stretch on your front hip as well as the workload for your core and legs.

- Hold a single weighted object, such as a purse, a briefcase or a frying pan, with both hands overhead.

- Hold two weighted objects, such as water bottles or paperweights, one in each hand overhead.

- Hold each lunge for more than 30 seconds.

> **TAKE 10 TIPS**
>
> Tightening your buttocks when holding the lunge position will help make your exits look as good as your entrances.

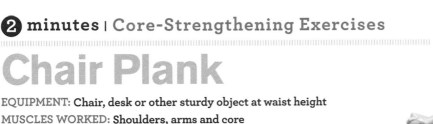

② minutes | Core-Strengthening Exercises

Chair Plank

EQUIPMENT: **Chair, desk or other sturdy object at waist height**
MUSCLES WORKED: **Shoulders, arms and core**

This exercise tightens your stomach, strengthens your lower back and hips, and creates a strong and healthy core without making you sweat. Even better, you don't have to get on the floor and perform a hundred sit-ups to make it happen. You can perform the Chair Plank anywhere—at home leaning against a washing machine or kitchen table, in the office leaning against the photocopier or outside leaning on a park bench.

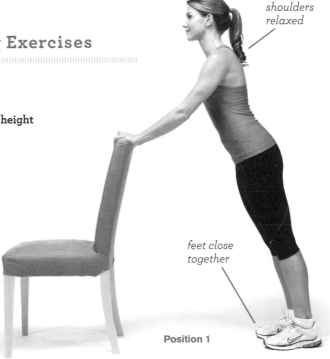

shoulders relaxed

feet close together

Position 1

▶ GET STARTED

Place your palms shoulder-width apart on a sturdy waist-high object. Next, walk 2 to 4 feet back. Keeping your feet close together, lean forward. This is your starting position. (**Position 1**)

▶ GET MOVING

1. Now imagine yourself as a long, strong board (or plank) leaning against a table. With your feet together and your upper body straight, and with your head in alignment with your body, rise up on the balls of your feet. Keep both arms extended, with a slight bend in both elbows. (**Position 2**)

2. Try to hold this position for 1 minute.

Too hard? Tone it down

- Walk closer to the object to decrease the weight on your upper body.
- Place your heels on the ground. When balancing your body is easier, the entire movement becomes easier.
- Hold the position for a shorter period of time.

Too easy? Kick it up

- Walk both feet farther away from the object to increase the weight on your upper body.
- Do a one-armed plank. Once you're in position, take one hand off the object for 30 seconds. Then switch arms for another 30 seconds.
- Do a one-legged plank. Tighten your abs, raise one knee toward your chest and hold that position for 30 seconds. Switch legs and hold that position for another 30 seconds.
- Hold the position longer than 1 minute.

TAKE 10 TIPS

To help you maintain proper head position, keep your head aligned with your body. To do your best plank imitation, keep your body tall and elongated and your abs tight.

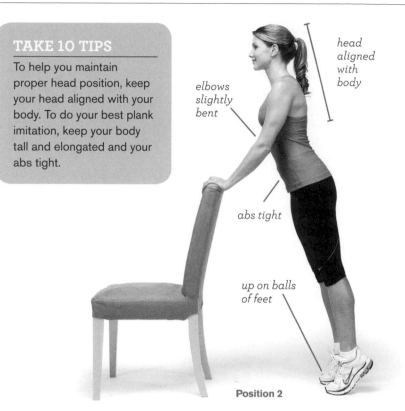

head aligned with body

elbows slightly bent

abs tight

up on balls of feet

Position 2

Chair Side Bend

EQUIPMENT: **Sturdy chair**
MUSCLES WORKED: **Core (abdomen, hips, lower back and sides of waist)**

Yes, you can tone and strengthen your abs and work on your waist while seated in a chair at work or home—even while watching TV! The Chair Side Bend is an easy exercise that provides you with the opportunity to train your core anytime, anywhere. It also serves as a wonderful lower back stretch.

❯ GET STARTED

Sit upright at the edge of a sturdy chair with your feet placed hip-width apart and your knees bent at a 90° angle. Make sure you're sitting firmly on the chair with your back straight. Place both arms straight at your sides with your hands below your waist. This is your starting position. (**Position 1**)

❯ GET MOVING

1. Begin by gently and slowly leaning your upper body to the left, lowering your left hand toward the floor, while keeping your buttocks positioned firmly on the chair. As you lean to the side, allow your head to move in alignment with your upper body. Tighten your abdominal muscles as you stay in this side-bent position for a count of 2 seconds. (**Position 2**)

2. Rise up to the original starting position and repeat the motion on the right side.

3. Perform as many repetitions as you can in 1 minute.

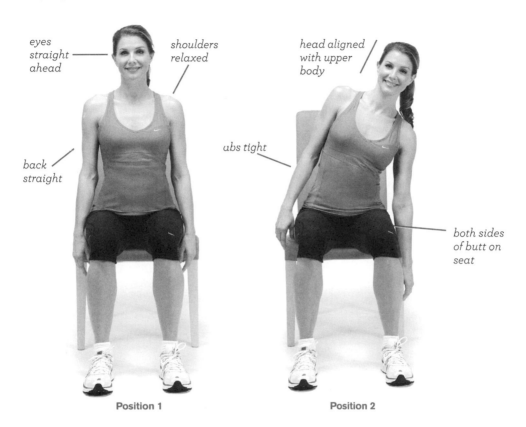

eyes straight ahead

shoulders relaxed

back straight

head aligned with upper body

abs tight

both sides of butt on seat

Position 1

Position 2

Too hard? Tone it down

- Decrease the distance you lean to the side. Instead of trying to bend as far as you possibly can, begin by leaning just a little bit and increasing inch by inch over time.

- Place your feet farther apart; this will increase your stability and balance.

- Hold the side-bend position for a shorter period of time.

Too easy? Kick it up

- Raise the opposite arm, as if you were asking a question in class. If you're going to lean to the left, put your right arm up straight. You'll feel the difference. This subtle change increases the difficulty of this exercise.

- Place your feet closer together. You'll be able to lean farther to the side, but you'll need to recruit more muscles if you don't want to fall out of your chair!

- Extend the opposite leg. If you're going to lean to the left, raise your right leg and hold it out straight. Keep your other foot on the ground. Then perform your side bend. This is another way of recruiting additional muscles. Alternate sides (and legs), and perform as many repetitions as you can in 1 minute.

TAKE 10 TIPS

To get the most out of this exercise, keep your shoulders relaxed and square as you lean over. Keep both sides of your butt firmly positioned on the chair. If one side seems to have a mind of its own, decrease the distance you are leaning. Rocking sideways defeats the purpose of the exercise. Keep your back as straight as you can.

1 minute | Stretching and Deep Breathing

Chair Forward Bend

EQUIPMENT: Sturdy chair
MUSCLES WORKED: Upper and lower back

How would you like to enjoy a relaxing back massage anytime you want? Well, the Chair Forward Bend is the next best thing. This gentle stretch works out the kinks in your back and provides soothing comfort to tight or sore muscles. By adding some deep breathing to this movement, you will increase the oxygen in your body and give your metabolism a boost.

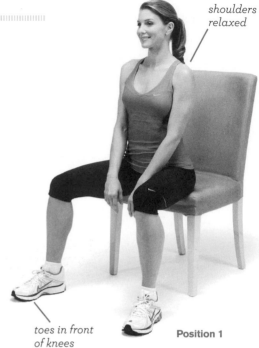

shoulders relaxed

toes in front of knees

Position 1

▶ GET STARTED

Sit upright at the edge of a sturdy chair with your feet placed firmly on the ground a little wider than shoulder-width apart. Bend your knees at a 90° angle so your toes are in front of your knees. Straighten your arms and place them between your thighs. Relax your shoulders. (**Position 1**)

▶ GET MOVING

1. Begin to bend forward from the waist. Lower your chin to your chest. Reach both hands down under the chair. Allow the weight of your upper body to pull you toward the floor. (**Position 2**)

2. Hold this position for 30 seconds, breathing deeply throughout this stretch.

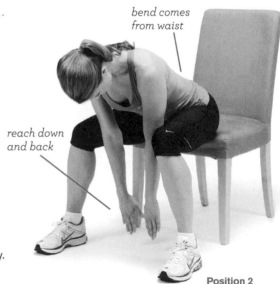

bend comes from waist

reach down and back

Position 2

Too hard? Tone it down

• Decrease the distance of the stretch.

• Allow your hands and arms to rest comfortably on top of your thighs as additional back support. When you're ready, slowly begin to lean down, bending from the waist, all the while using your hands and arms as support.

• Hold the stretch for a shorter period of time.

Too easy? Kick it up

• Place your feet farther apart and reach farther in the stretch position.

• Begin by placing your hands and arms outside your thighs. Relax your shoulders and elevate your chest as if you were sitting at attention. Slowly bend down as far as you comfortably can. Keep your head in alignment with your body.

• Hold the stretch for a longer period of time.

TAKE 10 TIPS

Do not "bounce" while you stretch, and do not push yourself until it hurts. Bend from the waist as you begin your stretch, allowing the weight of your head and upper body to help you. Breathe deeply, keeping in your mind the image of someone bowing—that's really what you're doing.

Chair Spinal Twist

EQUIPMENT: Sturdy chair
MUSCLES WORKED: Upper and lower back and sides of waist

"Make it with a twist!" means "Make it special." And special is how you'll feel after doing this gentle stretch.

› GET STARTED

Sit upright at the edge of a sturdy chair with your feet placed firmly on the ground hip-width apart. Bend your knees at a 90° angle. Cross your hands and arms over your chest "mummy style." (**Position 1**)

› GET MOVING

1. Twist your upper torso to the left, rotating from the waist and allowing your head and shoulders to move together as one unit. Rotate as far to the left as you comfortably can. (**Position 2**) Move slowly without straining or bouncing.

2. Hold this position for 15 seconds, and then repeat to the right for an additional 15 seconds.

Too hard? Tone it down
- Decrease the range of your stretch.
- Hold the stretch for a shorter period of time.

Too easy? Kick it up
- Raise your hands to shoulder level "zombie style" in front of your body before you begin your stretch. Rotate your upper body, leading with your arms. Remember to move your head in alignment with your upper body.
- Rotate farther in the stretch position.
- Hold the stretch on each side for up to 30 seconds.

TAKE 10 TIPS

To get the most out of this stretch, think of leading with your elbow as you turn your body to one side. Move your head in alignment with your body. Remember to breathe deeply! This helps significantly in your relaxation.

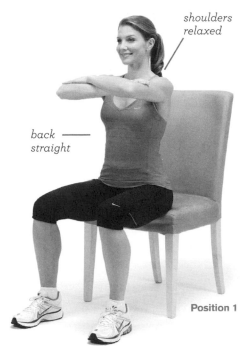

shoulders relaxed

back straight

Position 1

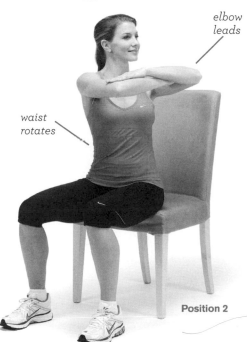

elbow leads

waist rotates

Position 2

LEVEL 1

Well done!
You did it! You completed your first 4•3•2•1 workout. Get a cool glass of water and give yourself a pat on the back. Or, for an extra challenge, go back and perform the whole circuit again.

WORKOUT 2

Here's another great workout that uses just your bodyweight. Like Workout 1, it can be done anywhere, anytime. Be sure to warm up first; if you don't have time, start with Marching in Place.

4 minutes | High-Energy Aerobic Training

Air Boxing and Marching in Place

EQUIPMENT: None

MUSCLES WORKED: Heart, shoulders, arms, core and legs

"Ding, ding! In this corner . . ." Today's H.E.A.T. exercise gives you the opportunity to be a prizefighter. And you receive all the benefits of a boxer's training—improving your fitness and endurance, and burning calories—while keeping your face pretty.

▶ GET STARTED

Stand with your weight on the balls of both feet, knees bent, with one foot behind the other. Next, make fists with both hands, being sure your thumbs are on the outside. Bring your fists up toward your face, at chin level. Pretend you're holding your fists up to guard yourself from being hit. This is your starting position. (**Position 1**)

▶ GET MOVING

1. While you exhale, throw your first punch. Extend your right arm in a jabbing motion in front of your body, knuckles on top. Keep your back straight and your knees slightly bent. (**Position 2**) Then bring your right fist back to its original position.

2. While you lean forward and exhale, throw your left fist out, punching the air in an uppercut, with your knuckles on the bottom. Raise your fist from waist level to head level. (**Position 3**) Then return your left fist to its original position.

3. Now do the same movements with opposite arms—a left jab and a right uppercut. Remember to exhale each time.

4. Continue alternating jabs and uppercuts with both arms for 30 seconds. Start gently, and progressively increase your intensity.

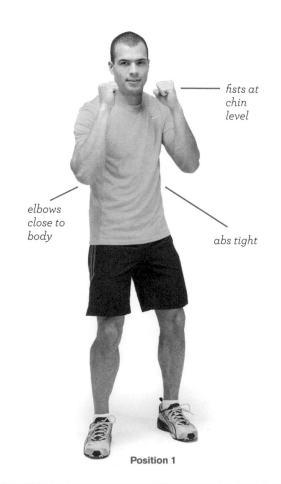

fists at chin level

elbows close to body

abs tight

Position 1

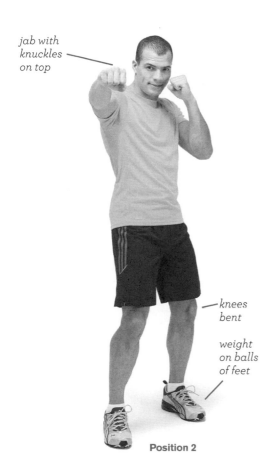

jab with knuckles on top

knees bent

weight on balls of feet

Position 2

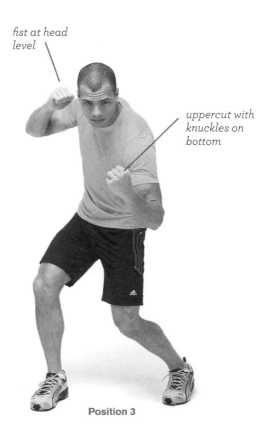

fist at head level

uppercut with knuckles on bottom

Position 3

5. Bring both arms down to your sides. Next, begin to march in place. Lift up your right knee while swinging up your left hand, and vice versa. Maintain a leisurely pace for 30 seconds.

6. Keep alternating moderately paced Marching in Place with rapid Air Boxing every 30 seconds, for a total of 4 minutes. See if your "slow" periods can progressively become just a little faster, and try to make your "fast" periods even faster.

Too hard? Tone it down
- Keep your hands on your hips while marching in place.
- Perform Air Boxing while seated in a chair.
- Punch more slowly.

Too easy? Kick it up
- Alternate between multiple jabs and uppercuts (throwing more than two of the same punches at a time).

- With each punch you throw, step in with the opposite foot.
- Bounce back and forth and side to side as you throw your air punches.
- Alternate between fast Air Boxing and slow Air Boxing instead of Marching in Place.
- Punch fast and explosively.
- Hold a water bottle or other weighted object in each hand.

TAKE 10 TIPS

As you air box, rock your weight back and forth until you find your rhythm. Remember to keep your abs tight. Grunting a little when you throw your punches will keep you focused and remind you to breathe.

LEVEL I

③ minutes | Resistance Exercise

Chair Squat

EQUIPMENT: Chair
MUSCLES WORKED: Legs, butt and core

The squat is one of the best ways to tone and strengthen your lower body, but if you do it wrong, it will put undue strain on your lower back and knees. As a trainer, I often resort to a trick of the trade: I place a chair behind my clients and ask them to sit down. Then stand up. Then sit down again, and then stand up. Over time, this simple motion of sitting down and standing up begins to train the muscles to move in the proper pattern. Next, I tell my clients to just gently "kiss" the chair with their butt, instead of sitting down, and then quickly stand up.

> **GET STARTED**

Place a chair behind you. Stand comfortably with your back to the chair, your feet shoulder-width apart. Keep your arms at your sides, your back straight and your chin parallel to the floor. This is your starting position. (**Position 1**)

> **GET MOVING**

1. Slowly lower your weight down, reaching back with your butt as if you were going to sit in the chair. Simultaneously raise both arms out in front of you to help you keep your balance as you descend into the squat. (**Position 2**) Go down as low as you comfortably can. Your goal is to touch the chair with your butt without actually sitting down.

2. Push back up to a standing position while tightening your buttocks.

3. In a slow and steady manner, complete as many repetitions as you can in 1 minute.

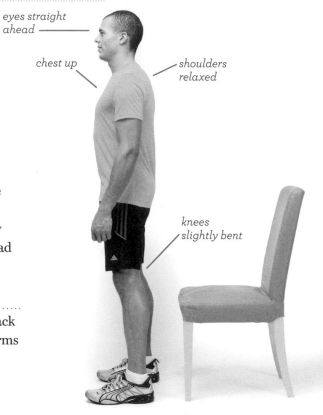

eyes straight ahead

chest up

shoulders relaxed

knees slightly bent

Position 1

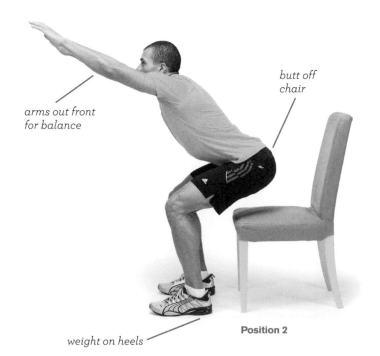

arms out front for balance

butt off chair

weight on heels

Position 2

Too hard? Tone it down

- Start with a quarter-squat.

- Keep your hands on your hips.

- Perform this exercise for less than 1 minute. Take a breather and then perform the Chair Squat again. It's okay to rest between repetitions.

Too easy? Kick it up

- Perform the squatting motion without a chair. This way you can descend lower.

- Perform the squatting motion with your arms over your head. Imagine you're making a "touchdown" signal with both arms straight up.

- Hold a single weighted object, such as a purse, a briefcase or a frying pan, with both hands overhead.

- Hold two weighted objects, such as water bottles or paperweights, one in each hand overhead.

- Quickly stand up as fast as you can when rising from the squat position.

- Hold the squat position for a longer period of time without sitting on the chair.

> **TAKE 10 TIPS**
>
> When you perform this exercise quickly, there is a tendency to bounce off the chair when rising up. Not a good idea! It's tough on your lower back and knees, as well as your body alignment.

Knee Push-Up

EQUIPMENT: **None (Optional: towel or exercise mat to cushion your knees)**
MUSCLES WORKED: **Chest, shoulders, arms and core**

When you were younger, was the dreaded push-up test part of your personal phys ed nightmare? Well, I'd like to take you back to school—not to torment you, but to teach you a push-up you can do well. The Knee Push-Up is your next step in learning to do a classic military push-up.

▶ GET STARTED

Lie face down on the floor in a push-up position, with your elbows bent. Your hands should be slightly wider than shoulder-width apart as well as slightly forward of your shoulders. While you're still lying down, with your thighs touching the ground, bend your knees at a 90° angle to form an L-shape. Now cross your ankles. This is your starting position. (**Position 1**)

▶ GET MOVING

1. Push both hands into the floor, extending your arms. Exhale as you push. Keep your back straight as your upper body rises. Keep your knees bent and your ankles crossed, with your head in alignment with your body. (**Position 2**)

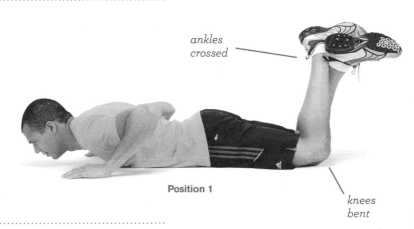

ankles crossed

Position 1

knees bent

LEVEL I

2. Next, tighten your abdominal muscles and lower your chest slowly toward the floor by bending both elbows. Go as low as you comfortably can. When performing this exercise, focus on keeping your thighs off the floor. Your only touch points to the floor are your knees and hands. The goal is to touch your chin to the floor without allowing your thighs to rest on the floor.

3. Being mindful of your form, do as many Knee Push-Ups as you can in 1 minute.

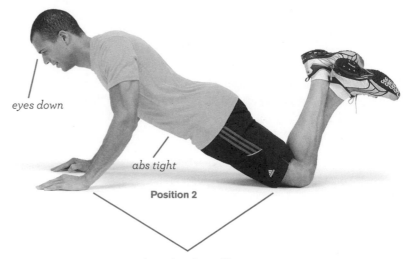

eyes down

abs tight

Position 2

weight on hands and knees

Too hard? Tone it down

- Go only a quarter of the way down as you lower yourself toward the floor. You don't have to touch your chin to the floor for this exercise to strengthen and tone the muscles of your upper body.

- Allow your upper thighs to rest on the floor.

- Go at your own pace and rest if you need to. As your muscles become better conditioned, you will increase the pace and the number of push-ups you perform.

Too easy? Kick it up

- Place your hands closer together in your starting position. This simple adjustment causes your triceps to work extra hard as you lower yourself into the starting position.

- Do a one-armed Knee Push-Up. Place one hand behind your back. Perform as many repetitions as you can in 30 seconds. Then switch hands for another 30 seconds.

- Do a one-legged Knee Push-Up. Uncross your ankles and extend one leg fully behind you without letting it touch the floor. Tighten your abs and transfer your weight to your other knee and your hands. Perform as many reps as you can for 30 seconds, then switch legs for another 30 seconds.

- Do push-ups explosively, pushing up as fast as you can.

TAKE 10 TIPS

The Knee Push-Up appears to be a very simple movement, but looks are deceiving. Form is everything! Keep your back straight, your butt down and your core strong throughout the entire exercise.

Forward Lunge

EQUIPMENT: None (Optional: chair or wall for balance)
MUSCLES WORKED: Legs, butt and core

You already mastered the Stationary Lunge. Now you get to take the lunge motion to its next progression, which involves repeating the lunging motion. This exercise tones and firms your entire lower body. You don't need any equipment, although I do suggest wearing a good pair of tennis shoes.

▶ GET STARTED

For your starting position, stand with your feet together, arms at your sides. Keep your chest up and look straight ahead. If you're using a chair or wall for balance, place one hand on the fixed object. (**Position 1**)

▶ GET MOVING

1. Step forward 3 to 4 feet with your right foot. Bend both knees, and lower your right thigh until it's parallel to the floor (or as close to parallel as you can manage). Balance your weight between the heel of your right foot in front and the ball of your left foot in back. (**Position 2**)

2. It's very important not to extend your right knee beyond the toes of your right foot. If this happens, try a longer stance and reevaluate the position of your front knee. You should be able to draw an imaginary vertical line from your front knee to the middle of your front foot.

3. Next, pressing from the heel of your right foot, push your weight back to your starting position, tightening your buttocks as you go.

4. Alternate sides, doing as many lunges as you can in 1 minute.

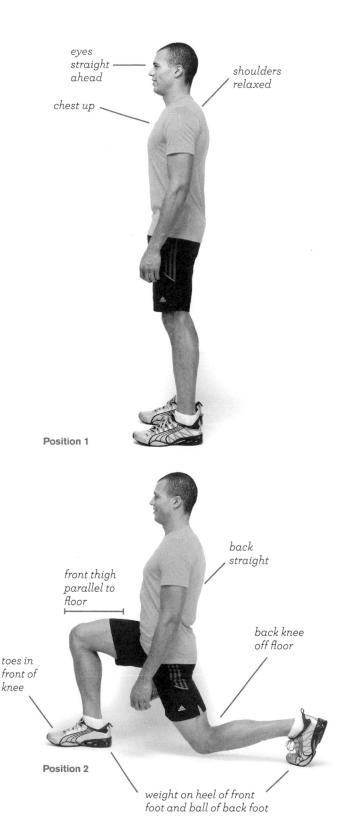

eyes straight ahead

shoulders relaxed

chest up

Position 1

front thigh parallel to floor

back straight

back knee off floor

toes in front of knee

Position 2

weight on heel of front foot and ball of back foot

Too hard? Tone it down

- Don't go so far into the lunge position. Instead of trying to lower your thigh parallel to the floor, begin with a quarter-lunge, bending your front and back legs slightly.
- Keep your hands on your hips.
- Rest between repetitions.

Too easy? Kick it up

- Go lower in your lunge.
- Perform the Forward Lunge on the same leg for 30 seconds, then switch to the other leg for another 30 seconds.

- Place your arms over your head. Imagine you're making a "touchdown" signal with both arms straight up. Keep your shoulders relaxed.
- Hold a single weighted object, such as a purse, a briefcase or a frying pan, with both hands overhead.
- Hold two weighted objects, such as water bottles or paperweights, one in each hand overhead.

> ### TAKE 10 TIPS
>
> Always adjust your stance to keep your front knee in alignment with the middle of your front foot. Look straight ahead and breathe comfortably throughout the exercise.

② minutes | Core-Strengthening Exercises

Reaching Ab Crunch

EQUIPMENT: **None (Optional: mat)**
MUSCLES WORKED: **Core**

For years, most trainers would tell their clients that if they wanted to tighten their abs they had to do lots and lots of sit-ups. But after years of fitness coaching, I can honestly tell you: There's a better way! The Reaching Ab Crunch is easy to execute and gives you a power-packed abs workout that does not put your lower back at risk. This exercise involves tightening your abdominal muscles as you reach for your knees and raise your shoulders off the floor.

If abdominal crunches are a priority for you, remember that you can do seated crunches anytime. In fact, you can perform mini ab crunches right now as you're reading this paragraph. All you need to do is tighten your abs as if you were protecting yourself from someone punching you in the stomach. Do this over and over and you'll feel them getting stronger.

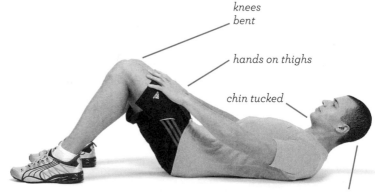

knees bent
hands on thighs
chin tucked
Position 1
head raised

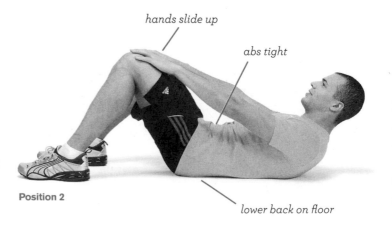

hands slide up
abs tight
lower back on floor
Position 2

❯ GET STARTED

Lie on your back on the floor with your knees bent and your feet hip-width apart. Straighten your arms and place your hands on top of your thighs. Now raise your head off the floor. Tuck your chin toward your chest as if you're holding an orange under your chin. (**Position 1**)

❯ GET MOVING

1. Tighten your abdominal muscles, exhale and raise your shoulders a few inches off the floor, sliding your hands up your thighs toward your knees as far as you can. Keep your lower back flat on the floor. (**Position 2**) Hold this position for 2 seconds.

2. Return slowly, touching only your upper back to the floor before quickly rising up again. Perform as many crunches as you can in 1 minute.

> **TAKE 10 TIPS**
>
> The correct form is to touch your upper back to the floor and immediately go right back up to another repetition.

Too hard? Tone it down

- Keep your chin tucked, tighten your abs and slide your hands up your thighs—but don't try to raise your shoulders off the floor.
- Between repetitions, lie on the floor and rest.
- Hold the upward position for a shorter period of time.
- Widen your stance. Placing your feet farther apart makes your position more stable, while bringing your feet closer together makes your position more unstable (making your muscles work harder).

Too Easy? Kick it up

- Fold your arms across your chest as you raise your shoulders off the floor.
- Place your hands behind your head. The best way to do this is to place your fingertips behind each ear. Do not lace your fingers together behind your head; this would cause you to pull on your head with your hands instead of making the muscles of your torso work harder.
- Hold the upward position for longer than 2 seconds.

Knee Plank

EQUIPMENT: **None (Optional: mat)**
MUSCLES WORKED: **Core, chest, shoulders and arms**

A great, no-sweat way to tone your abs, the Knee Plank strengthens your core as well as your chest, shoulders and arms. And you can do it anywhere!

❯ GET STARTED

Lie on your stomach on the floor, propped up on your elbows with your forearms and hands straight out in front of you and your legs straight out behind you. Your arms should be bent at a 90° angle so your shoulders are directly above your elbows. (**Position 1**)

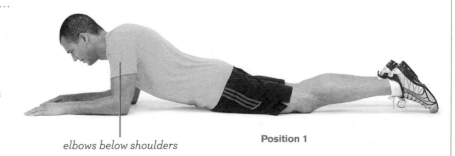

elbows below shoulders

Position 1

▶ GET MOVING

1. Raise your upper body and stomach off the floor, keeping your abdominal muscles tight. Your weight should be balanced on your knees, toes, forearms and elbows. Look slightly down, keeping your head in alignment with your back.

2. Next, slightly raise your hips (6 to 12 inches). Keep your back straight and your butt down. (**Position 2**) Hold this position as long as you can, up to 1 minute.

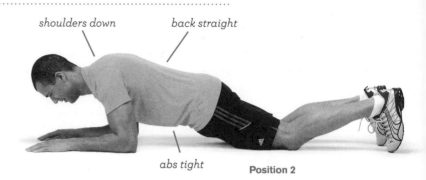

shoulders down   *back straight*

abs tight   **Position 2**

Too hard? Tone it down

• Hold the position for a shorter period of time.

Too easy? Kick it up

• Instead of placing your weight on your knees, raise your whole torso and balance on your elbows and the balls of both feet.

• Do a one-armed Knee Plank. Once you're in the Knee Plank position, lift your right elbow off the floor and extend your right arm in front of you. Balance your weight on your left elbow and your knees. Switch sides after 30 seconds.

• To make the above variation even more challenging, hold one arm behind you for 30 seconds, then switch arms for another 30 seconds.

• Do a one-legged Knee Plank. Once you're in the Knee Plank position, extend your right leg straight behind you on the same plane as your body. Balance your weight on your left knee and elbows. Hold this position for 30 seconds, then switch legs for an additional 30 seconds.

• Hold the stationary position longer than 1 minute.

TAKE 10 TIPS

Remember to tighten your abs throughout the entire exercise. Be sure to keep your back nice and straight and to breathe comfortably throughout.

① minute | Stretching and Deep Breathing

Chair Hamstring Stretch

EQUIPMENT: Sturdy chair

MUSCLES WORKED: Lower back and legs (hamstrings and calf muscles)

To stretch your lower back and hamstrings, here's an exercise you can do anytime you're sitting on a sturdy chair, on a park bench or even in your seat at a concert.

▶ GET STARTED

Sit at the edge of a sturdy chair. Bend your right leg at a 90° angle. Extend your left leg in front of you with your heel resting on the floor, and pull your toes up toward your shin. Rest both hands on top of your left thigh. (**Position 1**)

❯ GET MOVING

1. While keeping your chest up, your back straight and your head aligned with your torso, slowly bend forward from the waist. (**Position 2**) Do not tuck your chin into your chest, as this causes your shoulders to round. Breathe deeply and hold the stretch as long as you comfortably can, up to 15 seconds.

2. Switch positions (extend the other leg, bend the other knee, place your hands on the other thigh) and repeat for another 15 seconds.

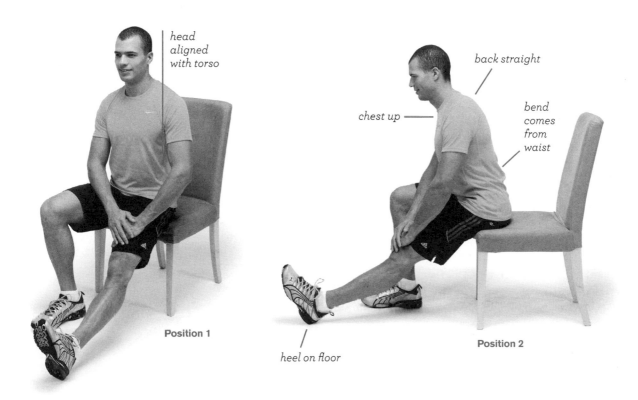

head aligned with torso

back straight

chest up

bend comes from waist

Position 1

heel on floor

Position 2

Too hard? Tone it down
• Decrease the depth of your stretch.
• Hold the stretch for a shorter period of time.

Too easy? Kick it up
• Descend farther in the stretch position.
• Hold the stretch for a longer period of time.

TAKE 10 TIPS

Remember to move slowly, bending from the waist and allowing the weight of your upper body to help you descend. Do not bounce or strain.

Chair Thigh Stretch

EQUIPMENT: Simple, sturdy chair without arms
MUSCLES WORKED: Fronts of legs (quads) and hips

It's time to get hitched! When describing this easy leg stretch to my clients, I often use the image of "proposing." Think of getting down on one knee to ask your loved one to eternally be yours. But this wonderful stretch comes without the butterflies in your stomach!

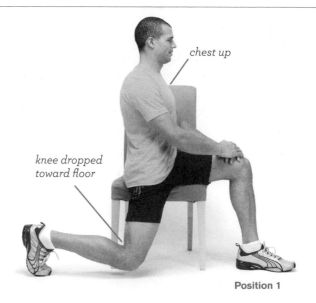

chest up

knee dropped toward floor

Position 1

▶ GET STARTED

Sit sideways on the edge of a chair with your feet placed firmly on the floor. Slide your body to the right so that you're sitting on your left buttock and your right leg is off the edge of the chair.

▶ GET MOVING

1. Keeping your chest up and your back straight, drop your right knee toward the floor without actually touching it, as low as you can comfortably manage. Keep your left leg bent at 90°, perpendicular to the floor. (**Position 1**)

2. Lean back slightly to stretch your hip and the front of your leg. (**Position 2**) Hold the stretch as long as you comfortably can, up to 15 seconds.

3. Switch sides and repeat with the other leg.

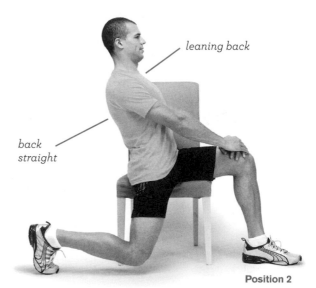

leaning back

back straight

Position 2

Too hard? Tone it down
- Don't lean back as far.
- Hold the stretch for a shorter period of time.

Too easy? Kick it up
- Lean back a little bit more to increase the stretch.

- Press the hip of your dropped leg farther forward as you stretch.
- Place your arms over your head. Imagine you're making a "touchdown" signal with both arms straight up. Keep your shoulders relaxed.
- Hold the stretch for a longer period of time.

TAKE 10 TIPS

Lean back slowly and with control, breathing deeply. Keep your back straight and your body elongated.

Way to go!
You have just completed your second 4•3•2•1 workout! Record your success in your journal. For an extra challenge, go back and repeat the entire workout or portions of it.

WORKOUT 3

They say three's a charm, and by the time you finish Workout 3, you'll be hooked on your new 4•3•2•1 exercise regimen. This workout is another step up the ladder to optimal fitness. You'll be pushing your body just a little bit more toward achieving your personal health and fitness goals.

4 minutes | High-Energy Aerobic Training

Jumping Jacks and Marching in Place

EQUIPMENT: **None**

MUSCLES WORKED: **Heart, legs, shoulders, arms and core**

The origin of the Jumping Jack is a toy with a wooden man on a string; when you pull the string, his arms and legs dance. If acting like a dancing puppet doesn't appeal, think of this exercise by the name it has in other countries: the Star Jump. Try to catch your own star! If you haven't had time to warm up, start with the Marching in Place movements.

▶ GET STARTED

Stand tall with your feet hip-width apart and your arms by your sides. This is your starting position. (**Position 1**)

▶ GET MOVING

1. Next, do two movements simultaneously. Jump up in the air and land with your feet 2 to 3 feet apart. Place your weight on the balls of your feet with your heels off the floor. At the same time, raise your arms above your head and place your hands in a clapping position. (**Position 2**)

2. Immediately jump back to the starting position, bringing your feet together and your arms back to your sides.

3. Start slowly to warm up. Progressively increase the intensity of your exercise until you're jumping up and down as fast as you can. Make sure your arms go all the way up with each jump. Keep up this pace for 30 seconds.

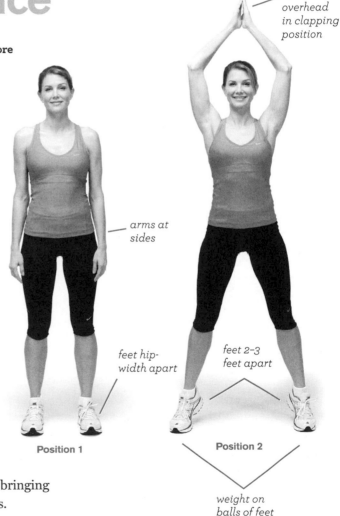

hands overhead in clapping position

arms at sides

feet hip-width apart

feet 2–3 feet apart

Position 1

Position 2

weight on balls of feet

4. After 30 seconds, bring both arms down to your sides. Begin your Marching in Place movements while standing. Raise your knees and swing your arms at a leisurely pace for 30 seconds.

5. Keep alternating slow-paced Marching in Place with fast-paced Jumping Jacks every 30 seconds for a total of 4 minutes. See if your "slow" periods can progressively become just a little faster and your "fast" periods can get quite a bit faster.

Too hard? Tone it down

- Perform Jumping Jacks in a chair. Use just your arms or incorporate your feet as well, all while sitting down.
- Keep your hands on your hips when doing your Marching in Place.
- Perform the Jumping Jack motions more slowly.

Too easy? Kick it up

- Do your Jumping Jacks faster.
- Alternate between fast Jumping Jacks and slow Jumping Jacks instead of Marching in Place.
- Hold a water bottle or other weighted object in each hand.

> **TAKE 10 TIPS**
>
> Select an area that has unobstructed room to jump high, plus flooring that provides some cushioning for your joints, such as a thin exercise mat or carpeting. Even better, go outside and jump on the grass. Have fun!

3 minutes | Resistance Exercise

Wall Slide

EQUIPMENT: **Wall or other fixed object**
MUSCLES WORKED: **Legs, core and butt**

This exercise is very similar to the Wall Squat, but now you'll be sliding up and down the wall. Be sure to wear shoes for traction, particularly if you're exercising on a slippery floor.

▶ GET STARTED

Lean your back against a smooth wall with your arms at your sides and your feet hip-width apart. Walk your feet out in front of you 2 to 3 feet. Bend your knees slightly. This is your starting position. (**Position 1**)

▶ GET MOVING

1. Look straight ahead, with your shoulders relaxed. Tighten your abdominal muscles, bend both knees and slide your back down the wall as low as you comfortably can.

2. If, during this exercise, you find that your knees extend beyond your toes, readjust your position by moving your feet farther away from the wall. When you're able to do a full wall slide, your knees will be directly over the middle of your feet. (**Position 2**) Hold for 2 seconds.

3. Next, pressing into the wall with your upper back and pushing from the heels of both feet, return to your starting position.

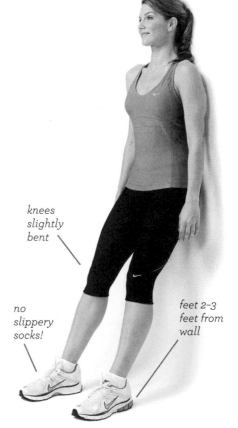

knees slightly bent

no slippery socks!

feet 2–3 feet from wall

Position 1

4. Slide up and down the wall as many times as you can for up to 1 minute.

Too hard? Tone it down

- Don't go so far into the squat. Start with a quarter-squat and then slide back up the wall.
- Keep your hands on your hips.
- Perform this movement for less than 1 minute.
- Take a breather between slides and start again when you feel rested.

Too easy? Kick it up

- Go lower into your squat.
- Place your hands over your head. Imagine you're making a "touchdown" signal with both arms straight up. Your thumbs should be pointed toward the wall and your palms facing each other. Keep your shoulders down.
- Do a one-legged Wall Slide. Once you're in the squat, slowly raise your left knee toward your waist, bringing your left foot a few inches off the floor. Transfer your weight to your right foot. To increase the challenge, raise your left knee higher. Perform wall slides for 30 seconds, then switch legs and continue for another 30 seconds.
- Hold a single weighted object, such as a purse, a briefcase or a frying pan, with both hands overhead.
- Hold two weighted objects, such as water bottles or paperweights, in each hand overhead.
- Perform this exercise for more than 1 minute.

TAKE 10 TIPS

I can't say this too often: Your knees should never extend over your toes when you're in the squat position.

eyes straight ahead

shoulders relaxed

chest up

abs tight

toes in front of knees

Position 2

Prowling Tiger Knee Push-Up

EQUIPMENT: **None (Optional: towel or exercise mat)**
MUSCLES WORKED: **Chest, shoulders, arms and core**

In this variation of the traditional military push-up, you alternate the position of your hands as if you were a tiger on the prowl. This employs different muscles from those used in the basic Knee Push-Up you performed earlier and takes your resistance training to the next level. It doesn't look especially challenging, but performed correctly it works every part of your upper body, with a lot of core involvement.

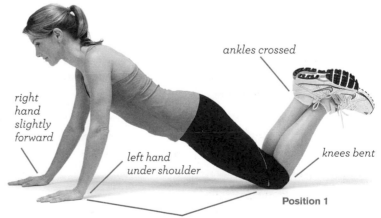

right hand slightly forward

ankles crossed

left hand under shoulder

knees bent

Position 1

weight on hands and knees

▶ GET STARTED

Lie face down on the floor in a knee push-up position with your elbows bent, but this time stagger your hands. Your right hand will be slightly in front of your right shoulder, next to your head, while your left hand will be directly underneath your left shoulder. While you're still lying down, bend your knees and cross your ankles. Now push up with your arms and raise your body until your weight is balanced on your hands and knees. Keep your knees bent and your back straight. This is your starting position. (**Position 1**)

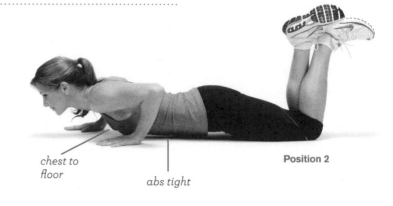

chest to floor

abs tight

Position 2

▶ GET MOVING

1. Bend both elbows and lower your upper body slowly to the floor, going as low as you comfortably can. Make sure your back stays straight and your butt stays down. Ideally, you will touch your upper body or chin to the floor. (**Position 2**)

2. Push against the floor with your hands and extend your arms. Exhale as you push your body back up to the starting position.

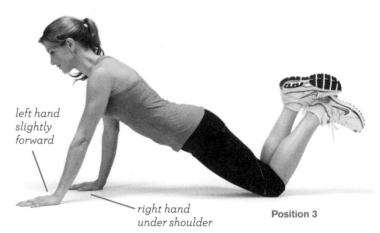

left hand slightly forward

right hand under shoulder

Position 3

3. Now shift the positions of your hands as if you were prowling. This time your left hand will be up next to your head and your right hand will be underneath your shoulder. (**Position 3**)

4. Alternating the positions of your hands between repetitions, do as many push-ups as you can in 1 minute.

Too hard? Tone it down
- Go down only a quarter of the way. Bend your elbows just slightly.
- Keep your thighs on the floor throughout the exercise.
- Don't stagger your hands as far apart.

Too easy? Kick it up
- Lower your upper body as far as you can.
- Bring both hands closer to the midline of your body.

- Perform push-ups explosively, pushing up as fast as you can.
- Do a one-legged Prowling Tiger Knee Push-Up. Uncross your ankles and extend one leg fully behind you without letting it touch the floor. Tighten your abs and transfer your weight to your other knee and your hands. Perform as many reps as you can for 30 seconds, then switch legs for another 30 seconds.

> **TAKE 10 TIPS**
>
> Keep your focus! Tighten your abs and keep your back straight throughout this exercise.

Backward Lunge

EQUIPMENT: None (Optional: chair or wall for balance)
MUSCLES WORKED: Legs, butt and core

Variety is the spice of life, so let me show you how to spice up the lunge. Here we step *back* into the position instead of forward.

▶ GET STARTED

For your starting position, stand with your feet together and your arms at your sides, looking straight ahead. (**Position 1**) If you're using a chair or wall for balance, place one hand on the fixed object.

▶ GET MOVING

1. Step backward 3 to 4 feet with your left foot, balancing your weight between the ball of your back foot and the heel of your front foot. (**Position 2**)

2. Lower your right thigh until it's parallel to the floor (or as close to parallel as you can manage). Next, lower your left knee toward the floor without actually touching it. (**Position 3**) It's very important

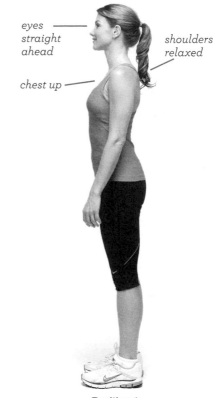

eyes straight ahead

shoulders relaxed

chest up

Position 1

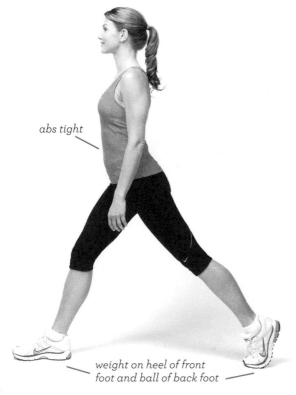

abs tight

weight on heel of front foot and ball of back foot

Position 2

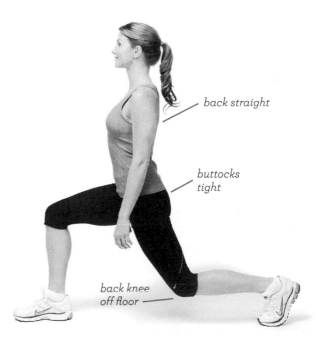

back straight

buttocks tight

back knee off floor

Position 3

117

not to extend your right knee beyond the toes of your right foot. If this happens, try a longer stance and reevaluate the position of your front knee. You should be able to draw an imaginary vertical line from your front knee to the middle of your front foot.

3. Next, pressing from the heel of your right foot and the ball of your left foot, push up and forward into your starting position.

4. Alternate sides and complete as many lunges as you can in 1 minute.

TAKE 10 TIPS

To get the biggest bang for your exercise buck, tighten your buttocks and press from the front heel.

Too hard? Tone it down
• Don't go so far down in the lunge position. Begin with a quarter-lunge, bending your legs slightly.
• Keep your hands on your hips.
• Rest between lunges.

Too easy? Kick it up
• Go lower in your lunge.
• Perform the Backward Lunge on the same leg for 30 seconds, then switch to the other leg for another 30 seconds.
• Place your hands over your head. Imagine you're making a "touchdown"

signal with both arms straight up. Keep your shoulders relaxed.
• Hold a single weighted object, such as a purse, a briefcase or a frying pan, with both hands overhead.
• Hold two weighted objects, such as water bottles or paperweights, one in each hand overhead.

② minutes | Core-Strengthening Exercises

Crossed-Arms Ab Crunch

EQUIPMENT: None (Optional: Mat)
MUSCLES WORKED: Core

Here's the next step in firming your abs. It resembles the Reaching Ab Crunch from Workout 2 (see page 108), but there's an added bonus. Check it out.

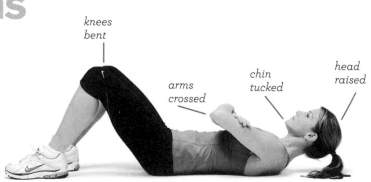

knees bent

arms crossed

chin tucked

head raised

Position 1

▶ GET STARTED

Lie on your back with your feet on the floor hip-width apart, and your knees bent. Place your hands and arms across your chest with your elbows crossed "mummy style." Raise your head off the floor and tuck your chin toward your chest as if you're holding an orange under your chin. (**Position 1**)

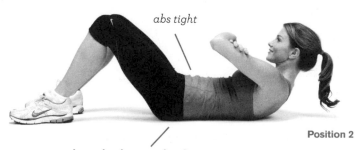

abs tight

Position 2

lower back pressed to floor

▶ GET MOVING

1. As you exhale, tighten your abdominal muscles and raise your shoulders off the floor just a few inches, raising your elbows toward the top of your knees. Keep the small of your back pressed to the floor. (**Position 2**) Hold this position for 2 seconds, then return slowly, touching your upper back to the floor and quickly rising up again.

2. Staying aware of your form, perform this movement as many times as you can in 1 minute.

Too hard? Tone it down
- Don't raise your upper back and shoulders as high off the floor.
- Lie on the floor between repetitions.
- Hold the upward position for less than 2 seconds.

Too easy? Kick it up
- Hold your arms out "zombie style" but with your palms facing each other.
- Hold the upward position for longer than 2 seconds.

TAKE 10 TIPS

Begin the crunch by tightening your abs as you raise your elbows up toward your knees and your shoulders off the floor. After going back down and touching your upper back to the floor, try to immediately go back up again.

Back Extension

EQUIPMENT: **None (Optional: mat)**
MUSCLES WORKED: **Upper and lower back**

Lying down on the job again? Now you have a good reason to do so. Here's a simple movement you can do at work, or home, or anywhere you can lie on your stomach. I know, I know—who's going to lie down at work and do this? Well, if you're someone who has back challenges or who wants to prevent them, I hope *you* will.

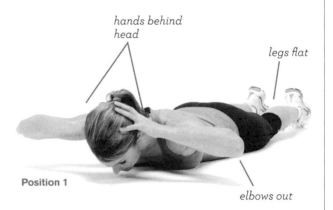

hands behind head

legs flat

Position 1

elbows out

▶ GET STARTED

Lie face down on the floor. Place your hands behind your head near your ears, with your elbows pointing out to the sides. This is your starting position. (**Position 1**)

▶ GET MOVING

1. As you exhale, raise your upper body off the floor by bending at the waist and pressing your hips into the floor. Lift up your torso as high as you comfortably can. Hold this position for 2 seconds. (**Position 2**)

2. Lower back down to your starting position.

3. Moving slowly, do as many back extensions as you can in 1 minute.

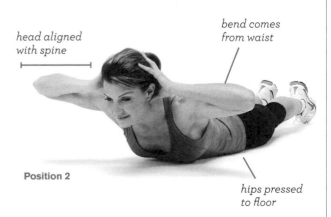

head aligned with spine

bend comes from waist

Position 2

hips pressed to floor

Too hard? Tone it down
- Place your hands at your sides, or behind your back.
- Hold the position for a shorter period of time.

Too easy? Kick it up
- Extend your arms straight out as you lift up.
- As you raise your chest off the floor, simultaneously raise one leg off the floor. Alternate legs.
- Hold the upward position longer than 2 seconds.

> **TAKE 10 TIPS**
>
> Be careful not to force your upper body up or to overstretch your lower back by pushing too hard. To get the most out of this movement, move your head in alignment with your spine—don't tuck your chin or throw your head back.

1 minute | Stretching and Deep Breathing

Standing Back and Hip Stretch

EQUIPMENT: **Sturdy chair or bench**
MUSCLES WORKED: **Buttocks, hips and back**

Ever play with a hula hoop? It's fun, right? Unless you're not so good at moving those hips. For most of us, hip flexibility decreases with age and sedentary living. This simple movement will get your hips working for you again. You don't need a hula hoop; all you need is a sturdy chair or bench.

> **GET STARTED**

Stand to the side of a chair seat or bench 18 to 20 inches high. Place your right foot on the seat, with your left foot planted firmly on the floor. Next, while bending from the waist, place your right elbow inside your right leg. (**Position 1**)

> **GET MOVING**

1. Bend forward farther from the waist, reaching your right elbow down toward your right heel. Reach down as far as you comfortably can. (**Position 2**) Move slowly without bouncing. Do not stretch to the point of pain. Breathe deeply throughout the exercise, holding the stretch as long as you comfortably can, up to 15 seconds.

2. Switch sides and hold the stretch for up to 15 seconds.

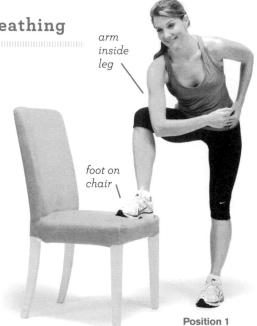

arm inside leg

foot on chair

Position 1

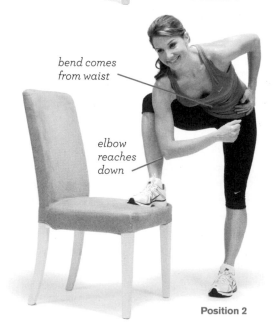

bend comes from waist

elbow reaches down

Position 2

Too hard? Tone it down
- Decrease the distance of your stretch.
- Hold the stretch for a shorter period of time.

Too easy? Kick it up
- Descend farther in the stretch position.
- Hold the stretch for a longer period of time.

Floor Spinal Twist

EQUIPMENT: **None**

MUSCLES WORKED: **Lower and upper back**

You've probably performed this movement many times before—but maybe not the 4•3•2•1 way. I want to show you how to do one of my favorite stretching motions correctly. Whenever your lower back is tight, sit on the floor and work out those kinks. You also can do a modified version of this stretch while seated in a chair (see the Chair Spinal Twist in Workout 1 on page 101).

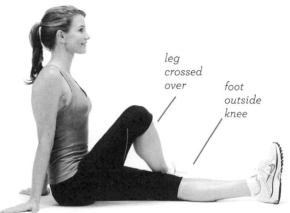

leg crossed over
foot outside knee

Position 1

▶ GET STARTED

Sit on the floor with both legs extended straight in front of you. Cross your right leg over your left. Position your right foot near the outside of your left knee. (**Position 1**)

▶ GET MOVING

1. Press your left arm against your right knee and thigh, pushing slightly, while rotating your shoulders, torso and head to the right as far as you comfortably can. (**Position 2**)

2. Hold the Floor Spinal Twist stretch as long as you comfortably can, up to 15 seconds.

3. Repeat on the other side. Cross your left leg over your right knee, press your right arm around your left knee, and twist. Hold the stretch for up to 15 seconds.

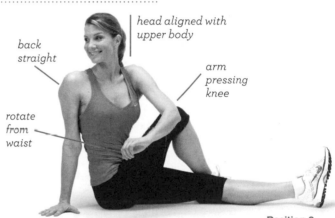

head aligned with upper body
back straight
arm pressing knee
rotate from waist

Position 2

Too hard? Tone it down
- Decrease the range of your stretch.
- Hold the Floor Spinal Twist for a shorter period of time.

Too easy? Kick it up
- Draw the foot of your bent leg farther up your thigh, toward your hip.
- Hold the Floor Spinal Twist stretch for a longer period of time.

Congratulations!
You have just completed your third 4•3•2•1 workout! You are becoming a pro at this stuff! Feel free to take a break, or go back and perform this same workout—or portions of it—again.

LEVEL I

WORKOUT 4

This is your last workout in Level I. Because the exercises in this workout use your bodyweight, you can perform them outside if you like. I want you to discover how much fun exercise can be when you change your surroundings. Here's hoping for good weather! If you haven't had time to warm up, start with slow-paced Marching in Place.

④ minutes | High-Energy Aerobic Training

High-Knee Marching in Place

EQUIPMENT: None
MUSCLES WORKED: Heart, shoulders, arms, core and legs

When I played football in high school and college, one of the most challenging exercises the coaches would make us do was high-knee running. They would stand with their hands on their hips, whistles in their mouths, intently watching (sometimes yelling) as we all tried to run through ropes or tires with our knees as high as they could go, over and over again for what seemed like an eternity. When I became a fitness coach, I knew high-knee running could be extremely beneficial for personal fitness, but there was a problem. The exercise is so demanding that it's tough to sustain for any length of time. Then one day, when I was watching a band move across a football field, I realized the musicians were doing high-knee *marching*. I found that marching in place as fast as I could, raising my knees as high as possible, was quite challenging. Try it. I won't be blowing my whistle.

▶ GET STARTED
Stand tall and erect with your hands on your hips. (**Position 1**)

▶ GET MOVING
1. Keeping your hands on your hips, start High-Knee Marching in Place by alternately raising your knees up toward your chest. (**Position 2**)

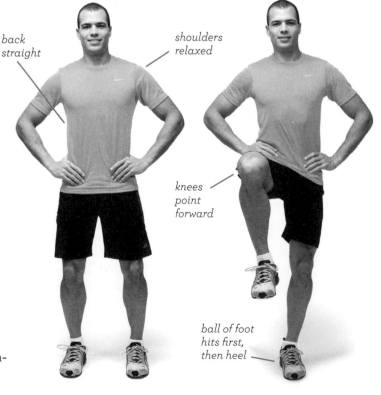

back straight

shoulders relaxed

knees point forward

ball of foot hits first, then heel

Position 1   Position 2

2. Start slowly, to warm up your body. Gradually increase the intensity, raising your knees higher and eventually as high and as fast as you comfortably can. Keep your hands on your hips. Be sure each foot strikes the ground in a rolling motion, first the ball of your foot and then your heel. Keep up this pace for 30 seconds.

3. Slow your pace down and begin Marching in Place. Swing your arms naturally, alternating legs and arms. (**Position 3**) Continue this leisurely pace for 30 seconds.

4. Keep alternating slow-paced Marching in Place with fast-paced High-Knee Marching every 30 seconds for a total of 4 minutes. See if your "slow" periods can progressively become just a little faster and your "fast" periods can get quite a bit faster.

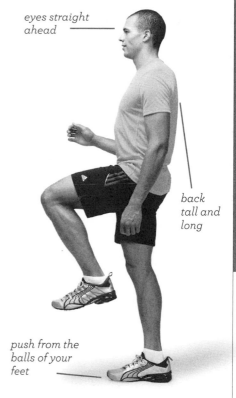

eyes straight ahead

back tall and long

push from the balls of your feet

Position 3

Too hard? Tone it down
- Do High-Knee Marching seated in a chair.
- Keep your hands on your hips when performing the Marching in Place exercise.
- Perform both exercises more slowly.

Too easy? Kick it up
- Move your arms along with your legs when you perform the High-Knee Marching exercise.

- Move your arms and legs faster.
- Hold a water bottle or other weighted object in each hand.

TAKE 10 TIPS

March in an area that provides some cushion for your joints—outside on some lush grass or inside in a carpeted area of your home or office. Now sign up for the band!

③ minutes | **Resistance Exercise**

Squat Thruster with Rotation

EQUIPMENT: **None**

MUSCLES WORKED: **Legs, core and butt**

The name of this exercise reminds me of a rocket! Now you'll be taking the squat exercise to the next level with a dynamic motion that involves both the upper and lower body. After you go into your squat, you will thrust your body back up and rotate your torso. This exercise is great for toning and firming your legs, core and butt.

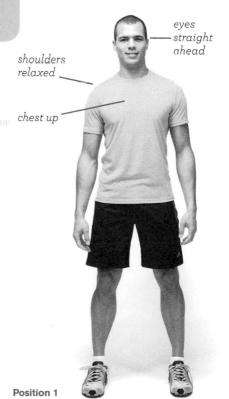

eyes straight ahead

shoulders relaxed

chest up

Position 1

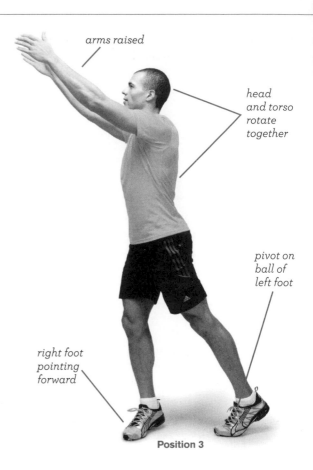

arms raised

head and torso rotate together

pivot on ball of left foot

Position 3

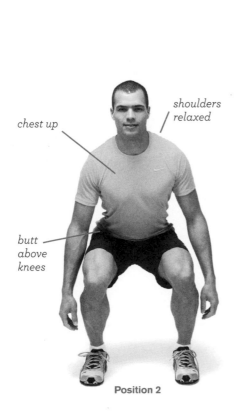

chest up

shoulders relaxed

butt above knees

right foot pointing forward

Position 2

❯ GET STARTED

Stand comfortably with your feet shoulder-width apart. Keep your arms at your sides, your back straight and your chin parallel to the floor. (**Position 1**)

❯ GET MOVING

1. With your arms at your sides, sit back into a squat position by slowly lowering yourself down as if you were going to sit in a chair. Go down as low as you comfortably can. (**Position 2**)

2. While you exhale, thrust your weight up as you raise both arms. While keeping your right foot pointing forward, rotate your head and upper body to the right. Pivot on the ball of your left foot, so your left heel comes off the floor. Keep your head aligned with your torso. (**Position 3**)

3. Bring your hands down to your sides and return to your starting position. Perform another squat, but this time, when you thrust back up, rotate to the other side. Keep your left foot pointing forward, and pivot on the ball of your right foot.

4. Continue doing squats, rotating to alternate sides, as many times as you can for up to 1 minute.

Too hard? Tone it down

- Don't go so far into the squat. Start with a quarter-squat.
- Hold the squat position for a shorter amount of time.
- Keep your hands on your hips.
- Take a breather between squats.

Too Easy? Kick it up.

- Go lower into your squat.
- Hold the squat position for a longer period of time.
- Increase your speed when coming up out of the squat and rotating.
- Hold a single weighted object, such as a purse, a briefcase or a frying pan, with both hands.
- Hold two weighted objects, such as water bottles or paperweights, one in each hand.
- Perform this exercise for more than 1 minute.

TAKE 10 TIPS

Squat Thrusters with Rotation are the most challenging squat exercises you have yet performed, and it's very important to do them correctly. Take it slow at first. As you become more comfortable with the motion, you can increase the speed of your thrust when you come up out of the squat.

Chair/Bench Push-Up

EQUIPMENT: **Sturdy chair, bench or solid object**
MUSCLES WORKED: **Chest, shoulders, arms and core**

Now that all those push-ups you've been doing have made your upper body stronger, I'd like to show you how to perform a push-up using a solid object such as the back of a sturdy office chair, park bench or couch at home. This exercise even works in a crowded airport if you find yourself waiting next to a sturdy waist-high barrier. The Chair/Bench Push-Up works the same muscle groups as the classic military push-up, but you don't have to do it lying down.

▶ GET STARTED

Find a chair or bench and assume a push-up position. Lean against the back of the object as you walk your feet 3 to 4 feet back. Place your hands shoulder-width apart, with your arms extended and your elbows slightly bent. Keep your back straight, and your legs almost straight with just a slight bend in the knees. Lift your heels so your weight is on the balls of your feet. (**Position 1**) Remember to keep your head in alignment with your back.

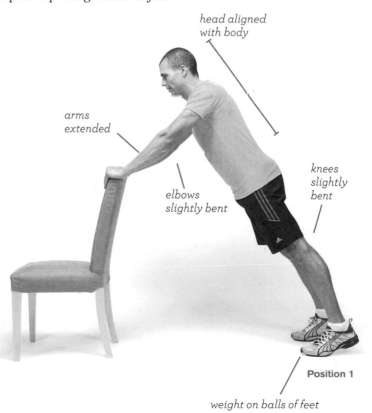

head aligned with body

arms extended

elbows slightly bent

knees slightly bent

Position 1

weight on balls of feet

LEVEL I

❯ GET MOVING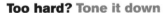

1. While looking down and slightly in front, lower your upper body slowly by bending both elbows. Go as low as you comfortably can. (**Position 2**) Aim your chest to touch the top of the object.

2. While exhaling, extend your arms and push your weight back to the starting position. Contract your chest muscles and the muscles at the backs of your arms, and keep your back straight and your core strong throughout the entire motion.

3. Do as many Chair/Bench Push-Ups as you can in 1 minute.

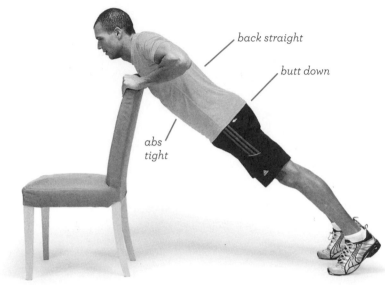

back straight

butt down

abs tight

Position 2

Too hard? Tone it down

- Go down only a quarter of the way. Bend your elbows only slightly.
- Stand closer to the object to reduce the weight on your arms.
- Take a rest between push-ups.

Too easy? Kick it up

- Lower your upper body as far down as you can.
- Walk your feet farther away from the object to increase the weight on your arms.
- Bring your hands closer together, underneath your chest. This will challenge the arm muscles more as you do your push-ups.

- After each push-up, hold your position for 2 seconds using one arm. Here's how: After you extend your arms and return to your starting position, raise one hand off the object and place it out in front of you. This will engage your abs. Alternate arms with each push-up. Perform as many repetitions as you can, alternating arms, in 1 minute. Be sure to keep your weight on the balls of your feet.

- Do a one-legged push-up. When you're in your starting position, raise one leg and extend it directly behind you as if you were a donkey kicking someone behind you. Perform as many reps as you can for 30 seconds, then switch legs and perform as many as you can for an additional 30 seconds.

- Perform your push-ups explosively.

TAKE 10 TIPS

Be sure to move slowly and under control throughout this entire motion, inhaling as you lower your upper body down toward the fixed object and exhaling as you push back to the starting position.

Walking Lunge

EQUIPMENT: **None**

MUSCLES WORKED: **Legs and butt**

Now that you've mastered the lunge, you're ready to take on the Walking Lunge. When it comes to toning and strengthening your lower body, nothing beats this exercise. It's simple to do, and it affects all the major muscles of your lower body. Best of all, you can perform it almost anywhere—all you need is a little room to move.

▶ GET STARTED

Stand with your feet together, arms at your sides. Keep your chest up with your shoulders relaxed, and look straight ahead. (**Position 1**)

▶ GET MOVING

1. Step forward 3 to 4 feet with your right foot. Balance your weight between the heel of your right foot in front and the ball of your left foot in back. (**Position 2**) (To review the Forward Lunge, see page 107.)

2. Next, lower your right thigh until it's parallel to the floor (or as low as you can manage). You should be able to draw an imaginary vertical line from your knee down to your ankle. Lower your left knee toward the floor without actually touching it. Looking straight ahead and keeping your back straight, balance your weight between the heel of your right foot and the ball of your left foot. (**Position 3**)

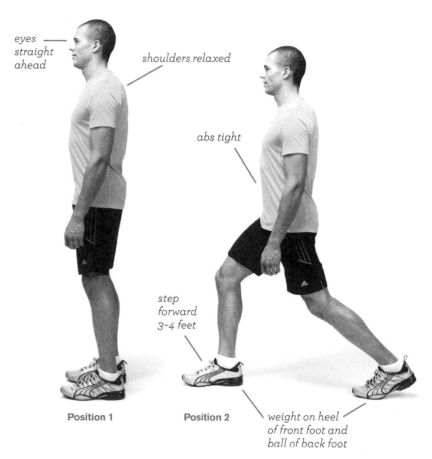

eyes straight ahead

shoulders relaxed

abs tight

step forward 3–4 feet

weight on heel of front foot and ball of back foot

Position 1   **Position 2**

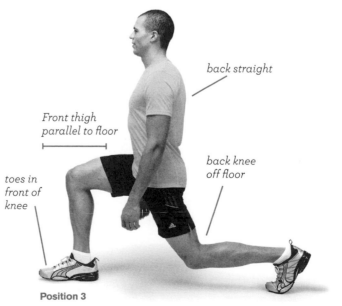

back straight

Front thigh parallel to floor

back knee off floor

toes in front of knee

Position 3

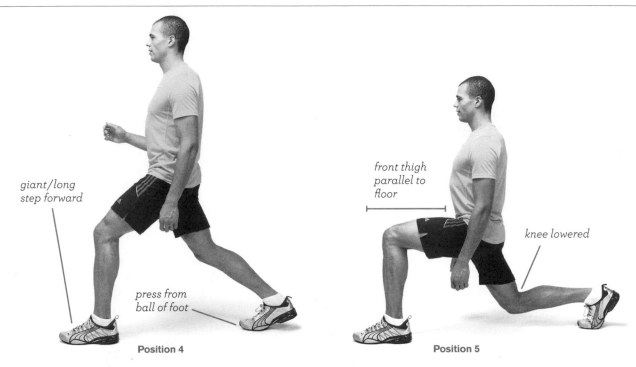

giant/long step forward

front thigh parallel to floor

knee lowered

press from ball of foot

Position 4

Position 5

3. Now walk into a lunge with your left leg. Take a giant step forward with your left leg by pressing from the heel of your front foot and the ball of your back foot. (**Position 4**) Lower your left thigh until it's parallel to the floor, and lower your right knee toward the floor without actually touching it. Remember to look straight ahead and to breathe comfortably. (**Position 5**)

4. Take another giant step forward with your right leg, into another lunge. Alternate legs and lunges as many times as you can for 1 minute.

Too hard? Tone it down

- Keep your hands on your hips.

- Don't go so far down in the lunge position. Instead of trying to lower your thigh parallel to the floor, begin with a quarter-lunge, bending your front and back legs only slightly.

- Rest between lunges.

Too easy? Kick it up

- Place your arms over your head as you lunge across the floor. Imagine you're making a "touchdown" signal with both arms straight up.

- As you transition from lunge to lunge, from leg to leg, raise the non-lunging leg up to your chest and stand on one foot for 1 or 2 seconds. Then continue your lunge motion.

- Go lower in your lunge.

- Hold a single weighted object, such as a purse, a briefcase or a frying pan, with both hands overhead.

- Hold two weighted objects, such as water bottles or paperweights, one in each hand overhead.

TAKE 10 TIPS

Congratulations! You have just completed an exercise of royalty. The king of lunges, the Walking Lunge will test your balance, strength and stamina all at the same time. Looking down can affect your balance, so remember to keep your eyes looking straight ahead.

2 minutes | Core-Strengthening Exercises

Back Bridge

EQUIPMENT: None (Optional: mat)
MUSCLES WORKED: Core, back, butt and legs

The Back Bridge works wonders—without any equipment!

▶ GET STARTED

Lie on your back with your knees bent and your feet on the floor hip-width apart. Place your arms next to your sides with your palms down. This is your starting position. (**Position 1**)

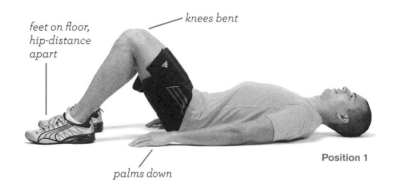

feet on floor, hip-distance apart
knees bent
palms down
Position 1

▶ GET MOVING

1. While exhaling, tighten your butt muscles and raise your hips 6 to 12 inches off the floor. Hold this elevated position for 2 to 5 seconds. (**Position 2**)

2. Return to your starting position and repeat. Don't lie down; just touch your butt to the floor and then immediately go right back up again.

3. Perform this movement as many times as you can in 1 minute.

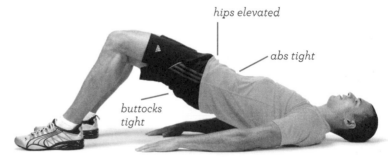

hips elevated
abs tight
buttocks tight
Position 2

Too hard? Tone it down
• Don't raise your hips as high.
• Rest on the floor between repetitions.
• Hold your hips up for a shorter period of time.

Too easy? Kick it up
• When raising your hips, raise one knee toward your chest.
• When raising your hips, straighten one leg and hold it off the floor.
• Hold up your hips for longer than 5 seconds.
• Perform this exercise longer than 1 minute.

TAKE 10 TIPS

To get the most out of this highly effective exercise, tighten your butt muscles and contract your abs as you raise your hips.

Side Bridge

EQUIPMENT: **None (Optional: mat)**
MUSCLES WORKED: **Upper and lower back, abs, sides of waist and hips**

Now that you've learned how to make a bridge on your back, here's an exercise that makes a bridge while you're positioned on your side.

▶ GET STARTED

Lie on your side, propped up with your elbow positioned directly under your shoulder and your forearm perpendicular to your body. Let your other arm rest on top of your body. Bend both knees behind you at a 45° to 90° angle. This is your starting position. (**Position 1**)

▶ GET MOVING

1. While you exhale, raise your hips off the floor, balancing your weight on your forearm and bottom knee. Lift your hips as high as you comfortably can, trying to make a straight line from your head to your knees. Don't let your hips rotate forward. Hold this position for 2 seconds. (**Position 2**)

2. Slowly lower your hips back down to the starting position.

3. Do as many Side Bridges as you can on this side for 30 seconds, and then switch sides and repeat for another 30 seconds.

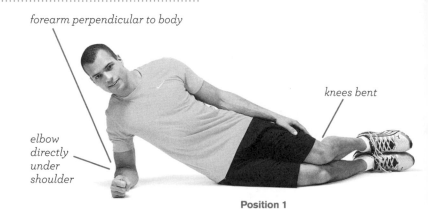

forearm perpendicular to body

knees bent

elbow directly under shoulder

Position 1

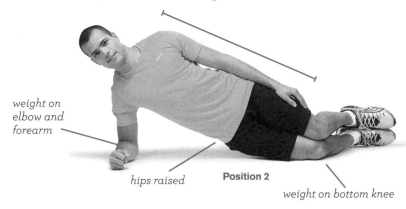

head, torso and knees in alignment

weight on elbow and forearm

hips raised

Position 2

weight on bottom knee

Too hard? Tone it down
- Don't raise your hips as high.
- Hold the position for a shorter period of time.

Too easy? Kick it up
- Instead of bending your knees, extend both legs and cross your ankles.
- Raise your top arm straight up.
- As you raise your hips, straighten your top leg and hold it about 6 inches off the ground.
- Hold the upward position for a longer period of time.

TAKE 10 TIPS

Focus on keeping your body straight, being careful not to swing yourself up in the air. Now you can say you've crossed that bridge!

1 minute | Stretching and Deep Breathing

Lunging Hip Stretch

EQUIPMENT: **None (Optional: chair or wall for balance)**
MUSCLES WORKED: **Hips, butt, legs, back and abdomen**

My daughter loves to play soccer, and I love to watch her and the other young athletes kicking a ball effortlessly but with precision. As a trainer and coach, I am amazed by how well they perform some of the game's most technical movements. One of the main muscle groups utilized in soccer, as well as in other sports involving running or kicking (or climbing hills or stairs), is the hip flexors. Individuals who are not competitive in sports often experience tightness in this area. If that describes you, the Lunging Hip Stretch will increase the range of motion in your back, hips and upper thighs. Even if you don't play sports, this stretch will help you be your best in the game of life.

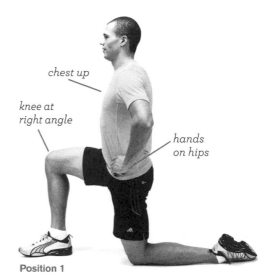

chest up

knee at right angle

hands on hips

Position 1

▶ GET STARTED

Position yourself on the floor, kneeling on both knees. Bring your right knee up as if you were proposing. Keep your left knee firmly planted on the floor. Place your hands on your hips. (**Position 1**)

▶ GET MOVING

1. Without moving your left leg, gently lean backward. (**Position 2**)

2. Hold this position for up to 15 seconds. Don't hold your breath!

3. Repeat on the other side, holding the stretch for up to 15 seconds.

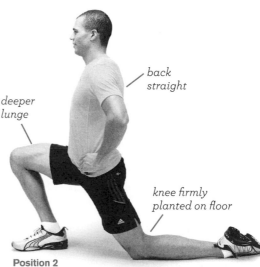

back straight

deeper lunge

knee firmly planted on floor

Position 2

Too hard? Tone it down
• Decrease the range of your stretch.

Too easy? Kick it up
• Lean backward to increase the stretch to your hip.

• Raise both arms straight up as if you're making a "touchdown" signal. Reach your hands high in the air to elongate your body and maximize the stretch.

• Hold the Lunging Hip Stretch for a longer period of time.

TAKE 10 TIPS

To get the most out of this stretch, slowly lean backward, all the while breathing deeply. Remember to keep your back straight and your body elongated throughout the motion.

Standing Side Bend

EQUIPMENT: **None**

MUSCLES WORKED: **Shoulders, upper and lower back and core (abs and waist)**

Asking a question can be good for your body as well as your brain. In this stretch, asking a question with the correct form can actually bring blood flow and flexibility to your shoulders, upper and lower back, waist and abdominal muscles.

▶ GET STARTED

Stand with your feet shoulder-width apart. Place your left hand on your left hip and raise your right hand as if you were asking a question in class. (**Position 1**)

▶ GET MOVING

1. Gently and slowly lean your upper body to the left, bending from the waist. As you lean to the side, move your head in alignment with your upper body. Your left hand stays on your left hip. Stretch to mild tension and hold. (**Position 2**)

2. Hold the stretch as long as you comfortably can, up to 15 seconds.

3. Repeat on the other side for up to 15 seconds.

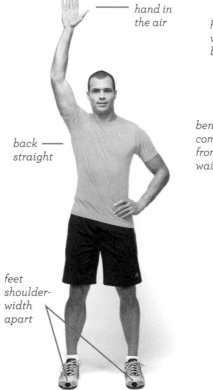

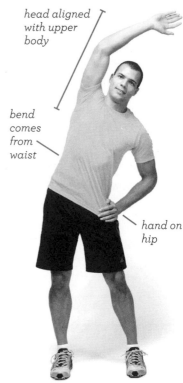

hand in the air

back straight

feet shoulder-width apart

Position 1

head aligned with upper body

bend comes from waist

hand on hip

Position 2

Too hard? Tone it down
- Perform the stretch while seated in a chair.
- Don't bend as far to the side. You'll increase inch by inch over time.
- Hold the stretch for a shorter period of time.

Too easy? Kick it up
- Increase the range of your stretch.
- Raise both hands over your head in a "touchdown" position as you perform the stretch. Keep your arms in alignment with your torso.
- Hold the stretch for a longer period of time.

TAKE 10 TIPS

Throughout this stretch, stand tall with your body elongated. Keep your shoulders relaxed as you lean to one side. In your eagerness to do a big stretch, don't let your upper body bend toward the ground.

Way to go!

You just completed your fourth workout in Level I! You can take a break and perform parts of the workout again, or repeat the whole circuit. Or you can have a party and celebrate how much you've accomplished this month! Complete the assessment on page 246 to determine how much your fitness has changed in the last month. Are you ready to go on to Level II? Or do you wish to repeat Level I, only making the exercises more challenging this time? Don't worry—either decision is the right one!

chapter 8

Level II: Moving On Up

Fitness Using Light Equipment

First, let me congratulate you on successfully completing Level I. That is a huge accomplishment, especially when you think about where you were just four weeks ago. Now you're ready to step up your workouts by adding more variety and by increasing the difficulty of your workouts. It's time to buy a few pieces of equipment: a jump rope, a resistance band and a stability ball. Using these items and the four new routines in this chapter, you'll get all the benefits of having more challenging workouts without the inconvenience or expense of going to the gym.

You'll be happy to know that putting together a home workout space is not expensive. It can be as simple or as impressive as you choose to make it. You may start out with a towel on the floor and a jump rope, or you may order top-of-the-line equipment for a home gym. As Lance Armstrong wrote, "It's not about the bike." What matters is your commitment to becoming the best possible version of you . . .

Working Out at Home or On the Road

Don't get me wrong. I think gyms are great. I've been a personal trainer in gyms my entire working life. I've made some amazing friends and have enjoyed the many advantages and amenities of fine fitness centers. But for most people, getting to the gym is just not realistic. So why not bring the gym to your home? All you need is a few portable pieces of exercise equipment and some clear floor space. Many of my clients travel a great deal and successfully exercise in their hotel rooms using the Level II workouts, so put a couple of workout items in your suitcase and you'll have your own traveling gym!

Convenience is not the only reason to do your exercising at home. Some people don't have the time (or child care) to get to the gym, or don't have the money to join. But for others an antipathy toward the gym may stem from fear (the machines *can* be intimidating) or shame ("Why is everyone else so fit?"). I'm going to encourage you to try the gym in Level III, but in the meantime focus on setting up a home exercise area. It will cost you $50 or less. If your car breaks down, the weather is bad or you can't find a babysitter, don't worry. You still can get in your 10-minute workout—and it will leave you feeling much better about your day.

Using some minimal gym equipment at home turned out to be the perfect solution for Andi, who's raising three daughters and wanted to set an example for them. "I struggled with weight my entire life," she says, "and I didn't want them to have to go through that. When I started 4•3•2•1, I loved the fact that I could just go downstairs and do my workouts!"

If You're Starting at Level II . . .

If you believe you're fit enough to skip Level I and start here at Level II, I strongly suggest that you first perform all four workouts at the end of Level I, using the recommendations to make all the exercises as challenging as possible. You may find that Level I is not as easy as you thought.

If you've completed the workouts in Level I at their most challenging and you're still convinced that you should start at Level II, then first read the list of ways to time your workouts (page 90), the intensity scale (page 91) and the information on warming up before each session (page 91). I also strongly suggest that you read the 28 days of daily instructions for Level I (starting on page 236) to get the full benefit of all the FUEL, RENEW and CONNECT tips.

Your Home Exercise Area

I know, right now you're probably thinking *"Gym equipment is so expensive!"* And you're right. Purchasing all the quality equipment for a home gym can cost thousands of dollars. But who says you have to buy all the equipment that gyms have in order to get fit?

You can begin without spending any money at all, although it would help to have around $50.

Take some time to evaluate your current budget and decide how much you have available to invest. Then figure out what you'll need for your home gym.

- **Decide on a space.** Find a location where you can safely perform your workouts. It could be anywhere in the house, garage or backyard; just make sure you have plenty of room to move. Consider things like the ceiling height, ventilation (windows or open doors are optimal) and the condition of the floor (a solid floor is best). If possible, choose a space where you can leave equipment set up. This will save time by allowing you to get right to your workout.

- **Determine what equipment you'll need.** I suggest starting out with a jump rope, some resistance bands and a stability ball.

- **Decide what amenities you need.** You may want to consider a television set, an oscillating fan and a boom box or stereo for music, as well as mirrors to check your form.

Suggested Equipment for Level II

With the equipment described below, you'll be able to master all of the workouts in Level II.

Jump Rope

If you own just one piece of cardiovascular equipment, it should be a jump rope. Jump ropes are very inexpensive and can be purchased at any major sporting goods store, usually for under $20.

You can get all the benefits of a full cardiovascular workout with this portable powerhouse piece of equipment. Jumping rope is one of the most comprehensive forms of cardiovascular exercise you can perform. It enhances your athletic ability and coordination, and expends more calories per hour than other aerobic exercises. It also tones your entire body, helping you achieve a lean look. Best of all, jumping rope is fun.

When shopping for a good jump rope, stand on the center of the rope and pull the handles up under your arms. The tops of the handles should reach your armpits. Before you buy, try a couple of jumps. If the rope doesn't touch the floor, it's too short; if it hits the floor in front of your feet, it's too long. (Don't worry if you're jump-rope challenged—you can simply hold both handles in one hand and pretend you're jumping over the rope. If even that has you worrying about tripping, don't buy one. When an exercise calls for a jump rope, just jump up and down and move your hands as if you were jumping rope.)

Resistance Bands and Door Attachment

At home or on the road, one of my must-have pieces of equipment is a resistance band. You can find one online or at most discount or sporting goods stores for under $15.

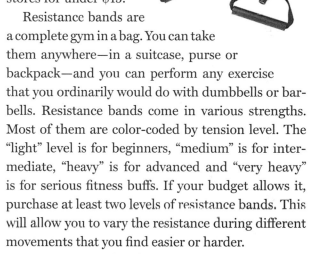

Resistance bands are a complete gym in a bag. You can take them anywhere—in a suitcase, purse or backpack—and you can perform any exercise that you ordinarily would do with dumbbells or barbells. Resistance bands come in various strengths. Most of them are color-coded by tension level. The "light" level is for beginners, "medium" is for intermediate, "heavy" is for advanced and "very heavy" is for serious fitness buffs. If your budget allows it, purchase at least two levels of resistance bands. This will allow you to vary the resistance during different movements that you find easier or harder.

Buy resistance bands with handles that provide you with a protective grip. I also suggest using a door attachment for your band; this unique product has a safety stop and provides a secure anchor for performing some of the exercises at this level. I recommend SPRI Xertubes, which are very high-quality and offer padded handles. We've used them successfully in our classes for years. Visit www.4321fitness.com to order directly from SPRI Products, a trusted partner store.

Stability Ball (Exercise Ball)

One of my all-time favorite pieces of equipment for stronger, healthier core muscles is the stability ball. You can find one online or at most sporting goods stores or discount stores for anywhere from $20 to $60.

Physical therapists and sports medicine doctors have used the stability ball for years for rehabilitation, and now fitness enthusiasts are catching on to its versatility and benefits.

The stability ball allows you to challenge your muscles without even realizing it. When sitting on the ball, your body is on an unstable platform, causing your muscles to contract just to keep you upright. When you couple this with a traditional exercise such as an arm curl or leg extension, your body has to work that much harder. The beauty of the stability ball is that you can perform almost any movement on it. From sitting on it at work to performing weighted exercises in a gym, it enhances your workouts dramatically.

Be sure the ball is the right size for you. When you get your stability ball, inflate it to the proper size. When you're seated on the ball, your hips should be even with your knees, nearly parallel to the floor. The chart below will help you determine which size is best for you, based on your height.

Size of Ball	Size of Ball	Your Height
55 centimeters	almost 20 inches	5' to 5'7"
65 centimeters	almost 26 inches	5'8" to 6'3"
75 centimeters	almost 30 inches	Taller than 6'3"

Some stability balls are better than others, so purchase yours from a reputable company. Visit www.4321fitness.com to order directly from SPRI Products, which offers quality stability balls at very reasonable prices.

Big-Ticket Equipment for a Cardiovascular Workout

Because treadmills and other cardiovascular exercise machines are so popular, you may want to complete your home gym by purchasing one of your own. These machines are usually expensive. It is not necessary to buy one for your home gym. Before you invest a lot of money in a treadmill or other expensive gym equipment for your home, see if working out at home is right for you. However, so many people enjoy the convenience of having their own exercise machine that I have included detailed information on my website to help you make the right choice. Before you purchase any large-ticket item like this, check out www.4321fitness.com for updates and information on the best buys, as we are constantly looking for the best fitness products in the marketplace.

Whether you're looking for a treadmill, elliptical machine, stationary bicycle, step machine or rowing machine, read the suggestions below to get started in the right direction.

Do your homework.	Do your research on a reputable website. Check with sporting goods stores and ask a lot of questions.
Try it before you buy it!	Take the time to go to your local sporting goods store or fitness warehouse and actually try some machines. Most stores are happy to oblige.
Take your physical limitations into consideration.	There are machines that allow you to work around problems like sore joints, a bad back or a trick knee. If you're very heavy or have back problems, try a recumbent bicycle.
Consider the "bells and whistles."	If high tech is your thing, then go for it, but it's not absolutely necessary for a great workout.
Get a machine with a good warranty.	Look for equipment that will provide you with a quality workout for many years without requiring much maintenance.

WORKOUT **1**

Welcome to your first workout at Level II. You are *moving on up* to the next level of fitness! By now, I hope you have purchased the only equipment you need for this level: a jump rope, some resistance bands and a stability ball. Like the 4•3•2•1 workouts in Level I, these four new workouts are designed to help you get fit and stay fit in minimal time. Each one will exercise every major muscle group, boost your energy level and metabolism, increase your strength and flexibility, and conclude with some stretching and deep breathing to help you unwind. Because they involve minimal equipment, you can do them not only in your home exercise area but anywhere you can find a little space—outdoors, in a hotel room, even at the office. To maximize your workout, remember to move quickly from one exercise to the next.

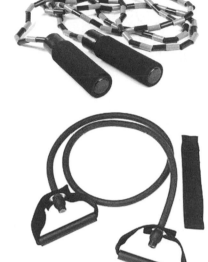

❹ **minutes** | High-Energy Aerobic Training

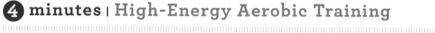

Jogging/Marching in Place

EQUIPMENT: None

MUSCLES WORKED: Heart, shoulders, arms, core and legs

If the word *jog* connotes pain, sweat and tears for you, I'm going to change your thinking by introducing you to a different form of jogging. Jogging is one of the best aerobic exercises; it improves your cardiovascular endurance, tones your muscles, boosts your energy level and metabolism, burns excess fat, relieves stress and keeps your "body age" young. When you perform the Jogging/Marching in Place exercise, you can get a good aerobic workout in a hotel room, at home or wherever you happen to be. You can control the surface on which you're jogging (for example, soft carpet instead of hard asphalt), you can wear whatever you want and you don't have to worry about traffic, pollution or cars honking at you. Best of all, you get all the benefits of jogging without having to turn around and come home! If you don't have time to warm up, start with the Marching in Place movements.

▶ GET STARTED

Stand tall with your chest up, shoulders relaxed, feet together and arms by your sides. (**Position 1**)

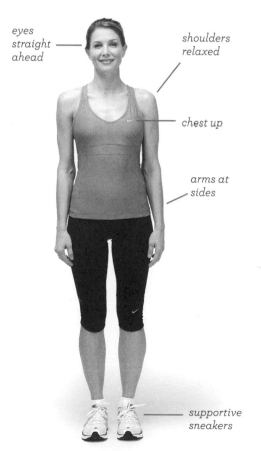

eyes straight ahead
shoulders relaxed
chest up
arms at sides
supportive sneakers

Position 1

❯ GET MOVING

1. Jogging comes first. Looking straight ahead, tighten your abdominal muscles and raise your right knee toward your chest, with your left arm driving up to your shoulder. Repeat on the other side. Remember to swing your hands all the way up. Keep your hands slightly open—no clenched fists. (**Position 2**) Be sure each foot strikes the ground in a rolling motion so you're pushing from the balls of your feet.

2. At first, go slowly to warm up. Jog at a moderate pace for 30 seconds.

3. Now begin your Marching in Place movements. Still looking straight ahead, raise your right knee toward your waist as high as you comfortably can. At the same time, swing your left arm up in a marching motion. Do the same on the other side. March in place at a moderate pace for 30 seconds. (**Position 3**)

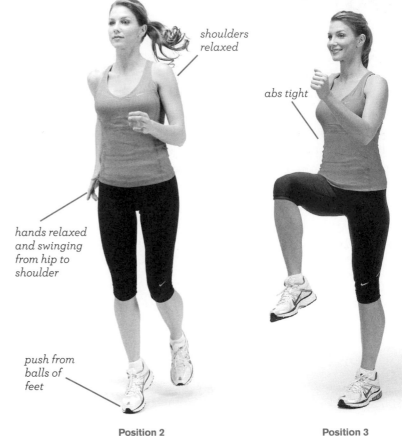

shoulders relaxed

abs tight

hands relaxed and swinging from hip to shoulder

push from balls of feet

Position 2

Position 3

4. Now return to jogging, but this time go faster. Keep alternating slow-paced Marching in Place with fast-paced jogging every 30 seconds for a total of 4 minutes. See if your "slow" periods can progressively become just a little faster and your "fast" periods can get quite a bit faster.

Too hard? Tone it down
- Keep your hands on your hips when marching in place.
- Jog more slowly.

Too easy? Kick it up
- While you're jogging, move your arms and feet faster.
- Alternate between fast jogging and slow jogging instead of marching in place.
- Hold a water bottle or other weighted object in each hand.

TAKE 10 TIPS

Choose an area that gives you some cushioning for your joints, such as a carpeted area of your home or some lush grass. Even if you're inside, wear sneakers to protect your joints. Remember to work both your upper and lower body. There you have it—no-hassle jogging!

LEVEL II

3 minutes | Resistance Exercise

Band Squat

EQUIPMENT: **Resistance band**
MUSCLES WORKED: **Legs, butt and core**

You learned how to do the Stationary Wall Squat in Level I, but a resistance band takes this exercise to the next level. Adding a little bit of extra resistance will help tone and shape your legs that much faster! Let me show you how it's done.

▶ GET STARTED

Holding your resistance band with a handle in each hand, place the middle of the band on the floor, then place both feet on top of the band shoulder-width apart with toes pointed slightly out. Keeping your knees slightly bent, position the handles at hip level. Now relax your shoulders and look ahead and slightly up. (**Position 1**)

▶ GET MOVING

1. Keeping your chest up, tighten your abdominal muscles and slowly lower your weight down into a squat position as if you're going to sit in a chair. Keep your hands and the resistance band handles at hip level. Remember that your toes should be in front of your knees. You should be able to draw an imaginary line from your knee to the middle of your foot. (**Position 2**) Go down as low as you comfortably can.

2. Next, tighten the muscles of your buttocks and push your weight up to a standing position, pressing from your heels.

3. While checking to make sure you're keeping perfect form, perform as many Band Squats as you can in 1 minute.

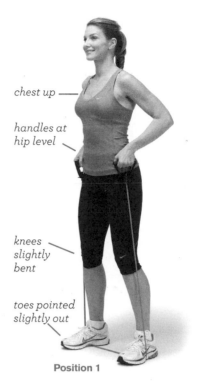

chest up
handles at hip level
knees slightly bent
toes pointed slightly out

Position 1

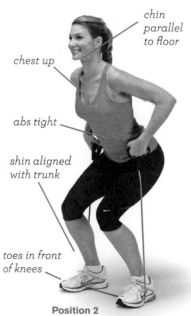

chin parallel to floor
chest up
abs tight
shin aligned with trunk
toes in front of knees

Position 2

Too hard? Tone it down
- Don't go so far into the squat. You can start with a quarter-squat.
- Choose a lower-level resistance band.
- Perform this exercise for less than 1 minute.
- Take a breather between squats.

Too easy? Kick it up
- Go lower into your squat.
- Each time you do a squat, hold it for a longer period of time.
- Hold the handles of the resistance band at shoulder level.
- Choose a higher-level resistance band.
- Perform this exercise for more than 1 minute.

TAKE 10 TIPS

Throughout this exercise, remember to breathe comfortably and to keep your back straight and your chin parallel to the floor.

LEVEL II

Band Press

EQUIPMENT: Resistance band and fixed object (door handle using door attachment or with door closed, or smooth pole, post or tree)

MUSCLES WORKED: Chest, shoulders, arms and core

Here's a great upper body exercise you can perform anywhere you'd like. All you need is a fixed object to wrap your resistance band around. Think of this exercise as a standing push-up. Over time, you'll be amazed at how toned and firm your body will become.

❯ GET STARTED

Find a fixed object to wrap your resistance band around. (Choose something with a smooth finish—a rough surface or a tree with a lot of bark will tear your band.) Loop the band around the object at waist to chest level. Turn your back to the object, and grasp a handle in each hand so that your palms are facing down. Keeping your hands at chest level, slightly wider than shoulder-width apart, bend both elbows at a 90° angle. The band should be running under both of your arms. Now that your arms are in position, keep your wrists strong and step forward 1 to 2 feet, increasing the tension on the band. Lean slightly forward, bending from the waist. Bending your knees slightly, place your feet in a staggered stance position, with your right foot forward and your left foot back. (**Position 1**)

❯ GET MOVING

1. Looking straight ahead, with your shoulders relaxed, tighten your abdominal muscles and push on both handles of your resistance band. As you exhale, extend both arms, keeping your elbows slightly bent, and bring your hands toward each other so that your thumbs come together. Tighten your chest muscles and hold this position for 2 seconds. (**Position 2**) Make sure your back is straight and your head is in alignment with your body.

2. Return to your starting position, keeping your arms and hands at chest level.

3. Perform this exercise as many times as you can in 1 minute.

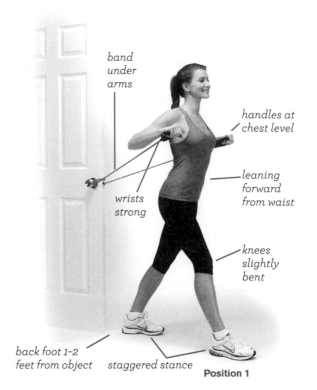

band under arms

handles at chest level

leaning forward from waist

wrists strong

knees slightly bent

back foot 1–2 feet from object   *staggered stance*   **Position 1**

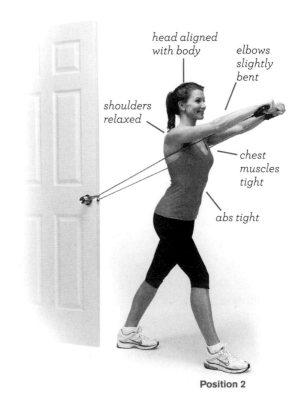

head aligned with body   *elbows slightly bent*

shoulders relaxed

chest muscles tight

abs tight

Position 2

LEVEL II

Too hard? Tone it down

- Back up, stepping closer to the fixed object. This reduces the tension of the resistance band.
- Bring the handles back only a quarter of the distance. You can bend your elbows slightly, then gradually increase the depth of your press as you become stronger.
- Choose a lower-level resistance band.
- Take a rest between repetitions.
- Perform this movement in a chair. (Choose a square-backed chair. If you use a rounded chair, the band may slip off and smack you in the back. Ouch!) Place the band around the back of the chair. Sit at the edge of the chair and lean forward, bending from the waist, then follow the instructions on the previous page.

Too easy? Kick it up

- Step farther away from the fixed object.
- Extend your arms and bring your hands closer together. If you wish, touch your hands together and hold.
- Do a one-legged Band Press. Raise your right foot off the ground, bringing your knee up to waist level and holding it there for 30 seconds. Switch legs for another 30 seconds.
- Choose a higher-level resistance band.
- Perform the Band Press explosively. By pushing the band handles away from you as fast as you can, you increase your total number of repetitions and also recruit more muscle fibers in your arms, chest and shoulders. Push out hard and fast, but bring the handles back to your starting position slowly.

> **TAKE 10 TIPS**
>
> Make sure your wrists are nice and strong throughout this exercise. Focus on keeping your back strong, abs tight and shoulders down and relaxed throughout the movement.

Band Lunge

EQUIPMENT: **Resistance band**

MUSCLES WORKED: **Legs, butt and core**

Using a resistance band takes the lunge to an entirely different level. Adding the tension of the band makes this exercise that much more challenging—and fun! This is an especially convenient exercise when traveling. All you need is your resistance band and a little space to get a great lower body workout.

> **GET STARTED**

Holding your resistance band with a handle in each hand, place the middle of the band on the floor, then step firmly with your right foot on top of the band. With your chest up and your shoulders relaxed, hold the band handles next to your hips. Next, step back 3 to 4 feet with your left foot. Looking straight ahead, evenly distribute your weight between the heel of your right foot in front and the ball of your left foot in back. (**Position 1**)

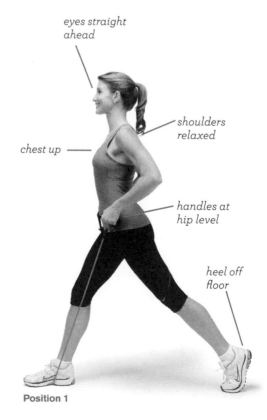

eyes straight ahead

shoulders relaxed

chest up

handles at hip level

heel off floor

Position 1

▶ GET MOVING

1. Assume the lunge position. Your hands, holding the band handles, will continue to stay at your hips. Keeping your back straight and your chin parallel to the floor, lower your right thigh until it's parallel to the floor (or as low as you can manage). With your abdominal muscles tight, bend your left knee down toward the ground without actually touching it. Balance your weight evenly between the heel of your right foot in front and the ball of your left foot in back. (**Position 2**)

2. Be sure not to extend your knee over your toes when in the lunge position. You should be able to draw an imaginary vertical line from your knee to the middle of your foot. If necessary, take a longer lunge step and adjust your stance to keep your front knee in alignment with the ball of your foot.

3. Still looking straight ahead, tighten your butt and leg muscles and push back to your starting position, pressing from the heel of your right foot in front and the ball of your left foot in back. Remember to keep your hands at your hips.

4. Keeping your right foot firmly on the resistance band, do as many Band Lunges as you can in 30 seconds. Now put your left foot on the band and do as many lunges as you can for another 30 seconds.

back straight

buttocks tight

toes in front of knee

Position 2

back knee off floor

Too hard? Tone it down

- Don't go so far down in the lunge position. Begin with a quarter-lunge, bending your front and back legs slightly.
- Rest between lunges.
- Choose a lower-level resistance band.
- Perform this exercise for a shorter time frame (for example, 15 seconds for each leg).

Too easy? Kick it up

- Place your hands and band handles at shoulder level instead of waist level. This change significantly increases the tension of the resistance band and the challenge of this exercise.
- Go lower into your lunge.
- Choose a higher-level resistance band.

TAKE 10 TIPS

As you do this exercise, move at a slow and controlled pace and remember to breathe comfortably. Don't look down—this can affect your balance.

② minutes | Core-Strengthening Exercises

Band Wood Chop

EQUIPMENT: **Resistance band and fixed object (door handle using door attachment or with door closed, or smooth pole, post or tree)**

MUSCLES WORKED: **Shoulders and core (abdominal, lower back and waist muscles)**

Tim-ber! Have you ever chopped wood before? If you have, you know it's one of the best ways to get your body in shape. For years, elite athletes have used actual wood chopping as a training method. When done properly, this motion works almost every muscle in your body. Now you will learn how to perform a simple but effective exercise that mimics chopping wood—without wielding a three-pound razor-sharp ax!

▶ GET STARTED

Find a fixed object to wrap your resistance band around. Loop the band around the object at a point at hip level or higher. Take a handle in each hand and step 2 to 4 feet away diagonally toward the left, creating tension on the band. Next, place your feet wider than shoulder-width apart, knees slightly bent. Now extend both arms, keeping your elbows slightly bent, so that you're holding both handles at the right side of your body (almost as if you were holding an ax). (**Position 1**)

▶ GET MOVING

1. Imagine you're chopping down a tree just in front of you. Holding your hands (and the band handles) close together, pull your arms and hands across the front of your body. Rotate your shoulders and hips to the left, away from the fixed object. While your left foot is pointing forward, your body will pivot on the ball of your right foot (the one closest to the fixed object) and your heel will be raised. (**Position 2**) Leading with your left shoulder, rotate until your torso is completely turned and your hands are on the left side of your body. Remember to move your head in alignment with your upper body.

2. Hold the farthest position for 2 seconds. (**Position 3**)

3. Slowly rotate back to your starting position.

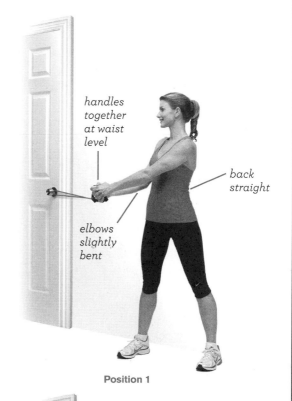

handles together at waist level

back straight

elbows slightly bent

Position 1

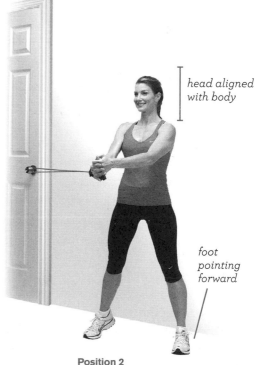

head aligned with body

foot pointing forward

Position 2

LEVEL II

143

4. Perform as many rotations to the left as you can in 30 seconds.

5. Now reposition yourself so that you're holding your hands on your left, pivoting on the ball of your left foot and rotating your torso toward the right. Complete as many rotations as you can in this direction for another 30 seconds.

Too hard? Tone it down

- Stand closer to the fixed object, decreasing the tension on the resistance band.

- Keep your arms bent throughout the entire exercise.

- Choose a lower-level resistance band.

- Perform the movement for less than 1 minute.

Too easy? Kick it up

- Step farther to the side of the fixed object.

- Move quickly and explosively when rotating away from the fixed object, but return to your starting position slowly.

- Choose a higher-level resistance band.

- Perform the movement for longer than 1 minute.

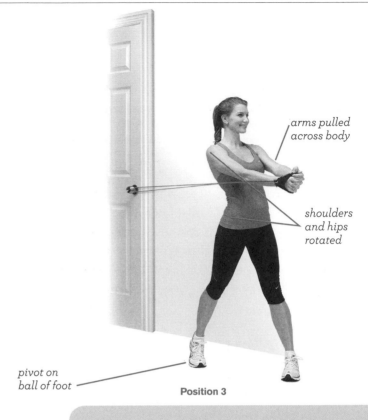

arms pulled across body

shoulders and hips rotated

pivot on ball of foot

Position 3

TAKE 10 TIPS

As you rotate your torso, allow your waist (oblique) muscles to initiate the Band Wood Chop motion, as opposed to swinging your arms down, generating the movement primarily from your shoulders and arms.

Standing Band Leg Raise

EQUIPMENT: **Resistance band**
MUSCLES WORKED: **Legs, hips and butt**

Want a lift? What if I were to tell you that you don't have to visit a plastic surgeon to get a good "butt lift"? The Standing Band Leg Raise helps lift the butt by strengthening the small muscle called the gluteus medius at each side of the hips. Let's take a moment to have a "butt-raising" experience!

▶ GET STARTED

Holding your resistance band with a handle in each hand, place the middle of the band on the floor, then place both feet hip-width apart on top of the band. Keeping your knees slightly bent, hold the handles at hip level. Relax your shoulders and look straight ahead, with your chin parallel to the floor. (**Position 1**)

❯ GET MOVING

1. Standing tall, shift your weight onto your left foot. Lift your right foot off the floor. Tighten your abdominal muscles and slowly raise your right foot as far as you can out to the side as you push against the band, beginning this movement at the hip. Both legs should be straight, but the knee of your left leg (the one that's not moving) should be slightly bent. (**Position 2**) Keep your head and back straight. Hold your position at the highest point, without changing your posture, for 2 seconds.

2. Slowly return your right leg to your starting position, without placing your right foot on the floor. Repeat the Standing Band Leg Raise to the right for up to 30 seconds.

3. Change legs and repeat the Standing Band Leg Raise to the left for another 30 seconds.

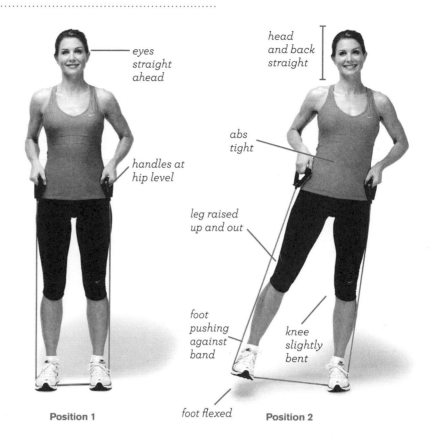

eyes straight ahead

handles at hip level

Position 1

head and back straight

abs tight

leg raised up and out

foot pushing against band

knee slightly bent

foot flexed

Position 2

LEVEL II

Too hard? Tone it down

- Choose a lower-level resistance band.
- Rest your foot on the floor between repetitions.
- Hold your raised leg in position for a shorter period of time.
- Perform the exercise for 15 seconds on each side instead of 30.

Too easy? Kick it up

- Hold the handles of the resistance band at shoulder level instead of waist level, close to your body.
- Hold your raised leg in position for a longer period of time.
- Choose a higher-level resistance band.
- Perform the exercise for longer than 1 minute.

TAKE 10 TIPS

This exercise is all about posture. Be careful not to bend to the opposite side as you raise your leg. Do not bend from the waist as you raise your leg, and don't let your shoulders dip down or lean to one side. Also, fight the tendency to drop your foot suddenly when you return to your starting position. You'll get much more out of this exercise if you move slowly on the way back. If you start feeling tired, think about how good your butt is going to look in your jeans!

① minute | Stretching and Deep Breathing

Hamstring Band Stretch

EQUIPMENT: Resistance band
MUSCLES WORKED: Backs of legs (hamstrings)

One of the best ways to alleviate lower back problems is to improve the flexibility of the hamstrings (at the backs of your legs). Let me show you a great way to stretch this area while lying on the floor. You can do the Hamstring Band Stretch anytime you have access to the floor—while you're lying in the middle of your living room watching your favorite TV show, for example, or by the side of your bed before you go to sleep or when you wake up in the morning.

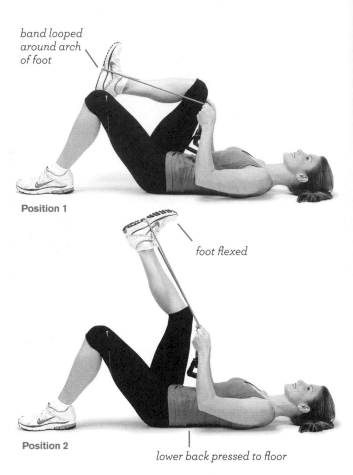

band looped around arch of foot

Position 1

foot flexed

Position 2

lower back pressed to floor

▶ GET STARTED

Begin in a seated position on the floor with both legs bent. Next, place the resistance band around the arch of your right foot with your hands grasping both sides of the band. Holding the band tightly with each hand, draw your right knee toward your chest and slowly lie down on the floor on your back. (**Position 1**)

▶ GET MOVING

1. As you're lying on your back with your head resting on the floor, slowly lift your right leg as straight as you can while maintaining a grip on the resistance band with both hands. (**Position 2**) Keep your left knee bent, with your left foot and lower back pressed to the floor. This will protect your lower back.

2. Hold the stretch for your right leg for 15 seconds. Then switch legs and hold the stretch for your left leg for another 15 seconds.

Too hard? Tone it down
- Don't try to straighten your leg all the way.
- Hold the stretch for a shorter period of time.

Too easy? Kick it up
- Pull down harder on the band.
- Straighten your leg more.
- Hold the stretch for a longer period of time.

TAKE 10 TIPS

Breathe deeply throughout this exercise, and avoid making any sudden movements. To get the most out of this stretch, remember to move slowly as you gently straighten your leg.

LEVEL II

Knees-to-Chest Stretch

EQUIPMENT: **None**

MUSCLES WORKED: **Upper and lower back**

I've read that we all need six hugs a day to experience optimal health. If hugging yourself counts, here's a great way to get your quota while at the same time stretching out your upper and lower back.

❯ GET STARTED

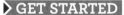

Lie on your back with your head resting on the floor. Now bring both knees as close to your chest as you can. Next, wrap your arms around (or hug) your knees and lower legs. (**Position 1**)

❯ GET MOVING

1. Gently pull your knees as close to your chest as you can. Squeeze your legs with your arms while pressing your lower back to the floor.

2. Stretch to mild tension and hold for up to 30 seconds. (**Position 2**)

Too hard? Tone it down
• Hold the stretch for a shorter period of time.

Too easy? Kick it up
• Hug your legs closer to your chest.
• Hold the stretch for a longer period of time.

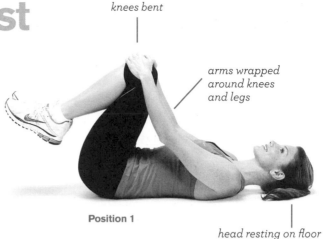

knees bent

arms wrapped around knees and legs

Position 1

head resting on floor

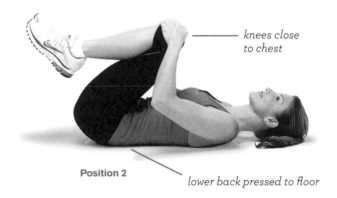

knees close to chest

Position 2

lower back pressed to floor

TAKE 10 TIPS

To get the most out of this stretch, remember to keep your head resting on the floor. Keep your lower back pressed to the floor as you gently pull your legs into your chest. Also, remember to breathe deeply as you give yourself a big hug. One down, five more to go—hugs, that is!

Way to go!
You just completed your first Level II workout! Now you can get back to your day—or, if you have time, go back and repeat parts of this workout or the entire circuit.

LEVEL II

WORKOUT 2

Are you ready to have a ball? In this workout, along with your resistance band you'll be using an inexpensive, versatile piece of exercise equipment that no home gym should be without: the stability ball. In a unique and powerful way, it helps you improve your strength, posture, cardiovascular endurance, flexibility and balance. Many of my clients buy one for their office and use it as a chair at work. Just sitting on it helps strengthen your abs and lower back. The stability ball is also a great piece of equipment if you have knee, back or hip problems. You'll discover that it takes certain movements to the next level, creating a greater impact on your upper and lower body as well as your core. In Workout 2, you'll learn techniques that combine multiple movements in one exercise to achieve fitness fusion— a proven way to maximize your fitness in minimal time.

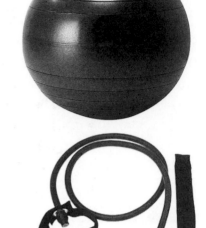

4 minutes | High-Energy Aerobic Training

Stability Ball Jog/Run

EQUIPMENT: **Stability ball**
MUSCLES WORKED: **Heart, shoulders, arms, core and legs**

> **GET STARTED**

How can you get all the benefits of sprinting, such as improving your cardiovascular system, toning and firming your core, and strengthening your arms and legs, without the wear and tear on your feet, hips or knees? By sitting down! The Stability Ball Jog/Run is exactly what it sounds like—you run as fast as you can while sitting on an exercise ball. This exercise is more challenging than you might realize, because you're sitting on an unstable platform, which forces your body to engage many different muscles. It's a great exercise to do when sitting down in front of the TV, when you're on a conference call at work— or, as I found out, even when you're typing a book!

> **GET STARTED**

Sit on top of your stability ball with your legs bent at a 90° angle, your feet hip-width apart and your toes in front of your knees. Look straight ahead, sit up tall and bend both arms at a 90° angle. (**Position 1**)

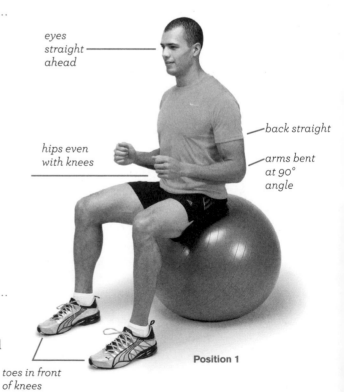

eyes straight ahead

back straight

arms bent at 90° angle

hips even with knees

toes in front of knees

Position 1

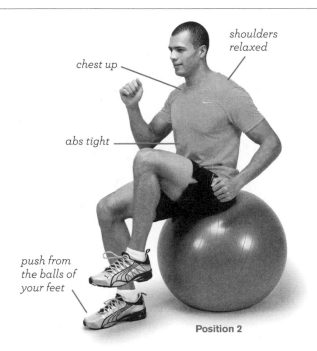

shoulders relaxed

chest up

abs tight

push from the balls of your feet

Position 2

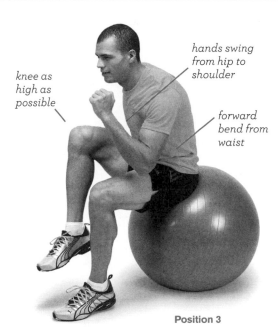

knee as high as possible

hands swing from hip to shoulder

forward bend from waist

Position 3

❯ GET MOVING

1. Tighten your abdominal muscles and begin to gently move your arms and legs in a slow jog. (This means your left arm and right leg go up at the same time, and vice versa.) Keeping your chest up and your shoulders relaxed, remember to raise your knees by pushing off from the balls of your feet. Jog at a leisurely pace for 30 seconds. (**Position 2**)

2. Now bend forward slightly from the waist and perform the same motions, but go faster. Run at a moderate clip for 30 seconds. Drive the balls of your feet down, and pump your arms and legs as fast as you can. Swing your hands all the way from your hips to your shoulders, and raise your knees as high as you can. (**Position 3**)

3. The first couple of minutes of H.E.A.T. are used to warm up, so ease into your workout, increasing your pace as you progress throughout the 4 minutes. Keep alternating slow and fast, every 30 seconds, for a total of 4 minutes. See if your "slow" periods can progressively become a little faster and your "fast" periods can get quite a bit faster.

Too hard? Tone it down
- Keep your hands on your hips or on the sides of the ball for balance throughout the movement.
- Move more slowly throughout the exercise.

Too easy? Kick it up
- Instead of alternating fast and slow, alternate intense and moderate.
- Move your feet as fast as you can while holding your arms straight over your head as if you were making a "touchdown" signal.
- Hold a water bottle or other weighted object in each hand as you run.

TAKE 10 TIPS

To get the most out of this exercise, keep your back straight—don't hunch over—as you pump your arms and legs as hard and as high as you can. If you feel unstable at any time, simply place your hands on the sides of the ball.

③ minutes | Resistance Exercise

Ball Wall Squat with Arms Raised

EQUIPMENT: Stability ball and wall
MUSCLES WORKED: Legs, butt, core and shoulders

The Ball Wall Squat with Arms Raised combines three movements into one power-packed exercise. It takes the Stationary Wall Squat (see page 93) and the Wall Slide (page 114) from Level I to the next level by adding an arm raise plus the challenge of using a stability ball to balance against. This exercise tones your entire lower body as well as your shoulders and can be performed anyplace where there is a wall. Athletes use this type of training to get the most out of their bodies. Now it's your turn!

▶ GET STARTED

Place the stability ball between you and the wall, positioning the ball at your lower to middle back. With your feet shoulder-width apart, 2 to 3 feet from the wall, lean against the ball and bend your knees slightly (don't completely straighten your legs or lock your knees). Relax your shoulders and place your arms by your sides. (**Position 1**)

▶ GET MOVING

1. Still leaning against the ball, tighten your abdominal muscles, bend your knees and slowly lower your body down into a squat as if you were going to sit in a chair. Allow the ball to roll down the wall with you. As you lower yourself down into the squat, extend both arms up over your head, elbows slightly bent, palms facing each other and thumbs to the wall. Go as low as you comfortably can. (**Position 2**)

2. Just as with a regular squat, your toes should be in front of your knees, and you should be able to draw an imaginary vertical line from your knee to the middle of your foot. If your knees are extended over your feet while you're in the squat position, move your feet farther out.

3. Next, pressing into the ball with your middle back and pushing from the heels of both feet, rise up to a standing position while lowering your arms back down to your sides.

4. Slide up and down the wall, raising and lowering your arms, as many times as you can for up to 1 minute.

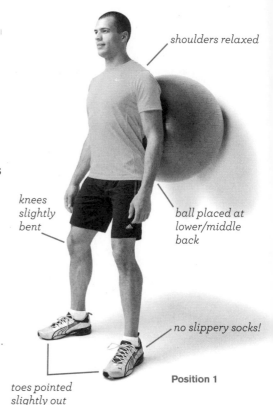

shoulders relaxed

knees slightly bent

ball placed at lower/middle back

no slippery socks!

Position 1

toes pointed slightly out

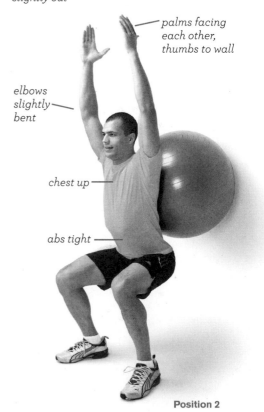

palms facing each other, thumbs to wall

elbows slightly bent

chest up

abs tight

Position 2

Too hard? Tone it down

- Start with a quarter-squat and slide back up the wall.
- Keep your hands on your hips.
- Perform this movement for less than 1 minute.
- Take a breather between squats.

Too easy? Kick it up

- Go lower into your squat.
- Do a one-legged Ball Wall Squat. Hold one foot off the floor for 30 seconds, then switch and hold the other foot off the floor for another 30 seconds.
- Hold a weighted object, such as a water bottle or paperweight, in each hand.
- Perform this exercise for more than 1 minute.

TAKE 10 TIPS

Remember to tilt your head slightly up, looking in front of you, and breathe comfortably during this exercise. As your leg strength improves, you'll be able to decrease the amount of pressure you maintain on the ball.

Seated Ball Band Press

EQUIPMENT: **Resistance band, stability ball and fixed object (door handle using door attachment or with door closed, or smooth pole, post or tree)**
MUSCLES WORKED: **Chest, shoulders, arms and core**

This exercise is like the Band Press in Workout 1 (see page 140) except that it combines a chest movement with a core-stabilizing exercise. Now you get double the fun!

▶ GET STARTED

Find a fixed object to wrap your resistance band around. Position your stability ball on the floor next to the fixed object. Wrap the band around the object at chest level. Holding both handles in one hand, sit down on top of the stability ball, facing away from the fixed object. Don't worry about positioning your feet yet. Next, holding a handle in each hand, place your hands on either side of the ball for stability and bend forward from the waist. This will increase the tension on the band. Continue to lean forward slightly and position your feet in front of you in a broad stance, wider than shoulder-width apart, to provide balance and support. Make sure your knees are bent at a 90° angle, so your toes are in front of your knees.

Now hold your hands up at chest level, slightly wider than shoulder-width apart, grasping a handle in each hand so that your palms are facing down and you're looking at the backs of your hands. Keep your wrists strong. The band should run under both forearms. Next, bend both elbows at a 90° angle. The band should be tight and straight, not loose or saggy. (**Position 1**)

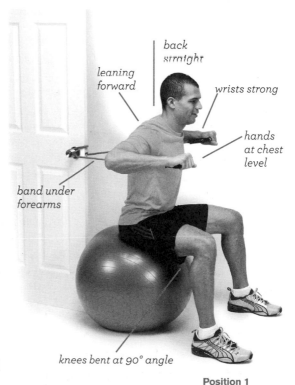

back straight
leaning forward
wrists strong
hands at chest level
band under forearms
knees bent at 90° angle

Position 1

LEVEL II

▶ GET MOVING

1. Looking straight ahead, with your shoulders relaxed, tighten your abdominal muscles and pull on both handles of the resistance band. As you exhale, fully extend both arms and bring your hands toward each other, bringing your thumbs together and keeping your elbows slightly bent. Tighten your chest muscles and hold this position for 2 seconds. (**Position 2**) Make sure your back is straight and your head is in alignment with your body.

2. Return to your starting position, keeping your arms and hands at shoulder level.

3. Repeat this exercise as many times as you can in 1 minute.

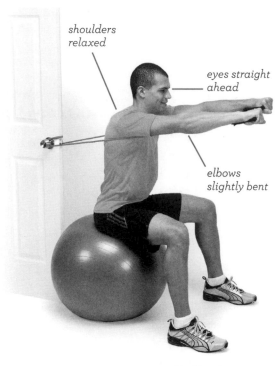

shoulders relaxed

eyes straight ahead

elbows slightly bent

Position 2

Too hard? Tone it down

- Roll back toward the fixed object to reduce the tension on the resistance band. Remember to reposition your feet correctly. You don't want to fall off the ball!
- Widen your stance for more stability.
- Bring your hands back only a quarter of the distance. You can bend your elbows slightly, then gradually increase the depth of your press as you become stronger.
- Use a lower-level resistance band.
- Take a rest between repetitions.

Too easy? Kick it up

- Roll the ball farther away from the fixed object to increase the tension on the resistance band. Remember to reposition your feet correctly.
- When you extend your arms, bring your hands closer together, touching your thumbs.
- Narrow your stance by placing your feet together as you balance on the ball. The more closely your feet are positioned, the more challenging this exercise becomes for your core.
- Do a one-legged Seated Ball Band Press. Raise your leg off the ground and extend it in front of you, holding it out straight while you keep doing band presses. Switch legs and continue for another 30 seconds.
- Choose a higher-level resistance band.

- Perform the band presses explosively. By pushing the band handles away from you as fast as you can, you increase your total number of repetitions and also recruit more muscle fibers in your arms, chest and shoulders. Push out hard and fast, but bring the handles back to your starting position slowly.

TAKE 10 TIPS

Remember to keep your wrists strong throughout this exercise.

LEVEL II

Ball Lunge with Band Shoulder Pull

EQUIPMENT: Stability ball, resistance band and sturdy wall
MUSCLES WORKED: Legs, butt, shoulders, upper back and core

Let's take it up to the next level! Now I'd like for you to experience a standing lunge movement combined with an upper body exercise using a stability ball and a resistance band. Wow! What a mouthful—but it sounds more complicated than it is.

▶ GET STARTED

To begin this movement, hold the stability ball with one hand and the resistance band with the other. Place the ball against the wall. Next, turn around and position your lower to middle to upper back against the ball. Now, step 2 to 3 feet forward with your right foot and place your left foot about 3 feet behind you, with your left heel near the wall. Balance your weight between the heel of your right foot in front and the ball of your left foot in back. This is the "split-stance lunge" position. Now lean against the stability ball by adjusting your front right foot. Be sure your right knee does not extend over the toes of your right foot. Remember to continue pressing back gently into the ball while in this position. Next, with both hands, grab the middle of the resistance band, pulling the band tautly, allowing the band handles to hang loosely next to your forearms and positioning your hands and arms a little wider than shoulder-width apart. Now extend both arms, with a slight bend in your elbows, and raise your hands and resistance band above your head with your palms facing away from you, and get ready for your Ball Lunge with Band Shoulder Pull. (**Position 1**)

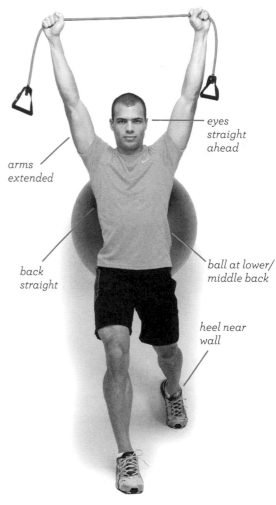

eyes straight ahead

arms extended

back straight

ball at lower/ middle back

heel near wall

Position 1

LEVEL II

▶ GET MOVING

1. Holding the resistance band above your head with your arms extended and elbows slightly bent, begin to pull the band "apart," bringing both hands down and out to the side while you simultaneously bend both knees, lowering your right thigh until it is parallel to the floor (or as low as you can manage) and lowering your left knee down toward the floor without actually touching it. You should be able to draw an invisible vertical line from your right knee to the middle of your foot.

Balance your weight between the heel of your right foot in front and the middle of your left foot in back. Hold this position for a count of 2. (**Position 2**)

2. Next, tightening your butt and leg muscles, return to your starting position by pressing from your right heel in front and the ball of your left foot in back and raising the resistance band with your hands and arms above your head.

3. Do as many repetitions of this exercise as you can in 30 seconds, then switch to the other leg and complete as many repetitions as you can for an additional 30 seconds.

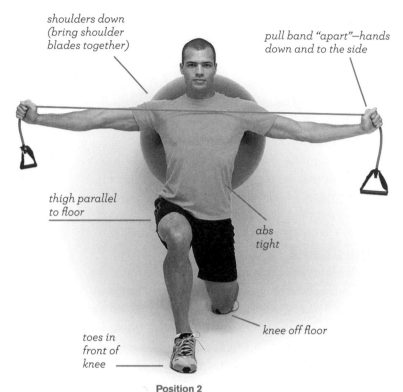

shoulders down (bring shoulder blades together)

pull band "apart"—hands down and to the side

thigh parallel to floor

abs tight

knee off floor

toes in front of knee

Position 2

Too hard? Tone it down

- Don't go so far down in the lunge position. Instead of trying to lower your legs to a parallel position, begin with a lunge, bending your front and back legs slightly.
- When holding the resistance band, hold hands farther apart. The wider your hands are when holding the resistance band, the easier the exercise.
- Rest between repetitions.
- Choose a lower-level resistance band.
- Perform this exercise for a shorter time period (e.g. 15 seconds per leg, then switch).

Too easy? Kick it up

- Go lower in your lunge.
- When holding the resistance band, hold your hands close together. The closer your hands are when holding the resistance band, the more challenging the exercise.
- Choose a higher-level resistance band.
- Perform the exercise for a longer period of time.

TAKE 10 TIPS

Do this exercise at a slow and controlled pace, breathing comfortably. With your back straight, keep leaning back into the stability ball. Remember to look straight ahead—looking down can affect your balance.

LEVEL II

② minutes | Core-Strengthening Exercises

Ball Ab Crunch

EQUIPMENT: **Stability ball**
MUSCLES WORKED: **Core**

Now it's time to take your crunches to the next level. By adding a stability ball to the abdominal crunch, you provide an extra dose of fitness fusion. You can do this exercise anytime you're in the mood to tone and strengthen your abs and back. The best part about these crunches is that, by modifying your hand placement and the angle of your feet, you can make this movement as easy or as difficult as you'd like.

▶ GET STARTED

Sit on top of the stability ball, then walk your feet forward, pressing your back and hips into the ball until your lower back is firmly supported by the ball and your knees are at a 90° angle. Press your feet into the floor and your back into the ball to keep the ball from moving. Next, place your feet a little wider than shoulder-width apart, flat on the floor, and extend your arms out on top of your thighs. Tuck your chin toward your chest as if you're holding an orange under your chin. (**Position 1**)

▶ GET MOVING

1. As you exhale, tighten your abdominal muscles and raise your middle/upper back off the stability ball, sliding your hands up your thighs toward your knees as far as you can while pressing your lower back/hips down into the ball. (**Position 2**) Hold this position for 2 seconds, remembering to tighten your stomach muscles. Then return slowly to your starting position, touching your middle/upper back to the ball.

2. Immediately go back up into another repetition.

3. Perform this movement as many times as you can for up to 1 minute.

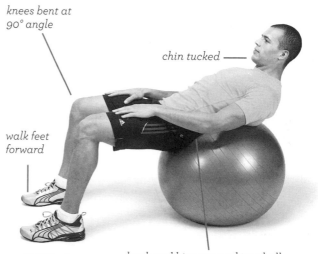

knees bent at 90° angle

chin tucked

walk feet forward

back and hips pressed into ball

Position 1

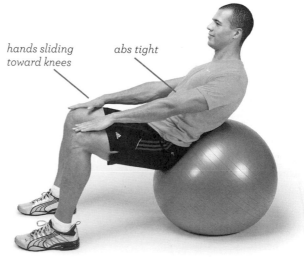

hands sliding toward knees

abs tight

Position 2

LEVEL II

Too hard? Tone it down

- Don't raise your back as high. Just tighten your abs as you slide your hands toward your knees.
- Hold the crunch for a shorter period of time.
- Rest between crunches.
- Perform this movement for less than 1 minute.

Too easy? Kick it up

- Change the position of your hands. Try folding your arms across your chest, or place the tips of your fingers behind your ears.
- Walk your feet back and sit farther back on top of the ball, exposing more of your middle back off the ball. The less back support you get from the ball, the more challenging the exercise.
- Place your feet closer together to make your position less stable and recruit more muscles.

- Do a one-legged Ball Ab Crunch. Raise one foot off the ground for 30 seconds, then switch legs for another 30 seconds.
- Hold the crunch position for longer than 2 seconds.
- Perform this movement for more than 1 minute.

> **TAKE 10 TIPS**
>
> Remember to keep your chin tucked and your abs tight throughout this exercise. Be patient—using the stability ball can take some getting used to.

Ball Balance

EQUIPMENT: **Stability ball**

MUSCLES WORKED: **Upper and lower back**

Professional athletes with lower back pain often come to see me for an exercise to get them back in action as soon as possible. The Ball Balance is the one I recommend—not only for professional athletes, but for all of us! This is a great exercise to strengthen your upper and lower back. It's very simple to perform and doesn't take much time, but it's highly effective.

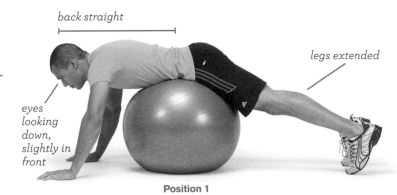

back straight

legs extended

eyes looking down, slightly in front

Position 1

▶ **GET STARTED**

Begin this exercise by assuming the position of a classic push-up—but with a stability ball under your hips. Lie down on top of the ball, placing your hands on the floor wider than shoulder-width apart and your feet on the floor wider than hip-width apart. Your legs should be straight out behind you, without your knees touching the floor. (**Position 1**) Now look down and slightly in front. You're ready to go.

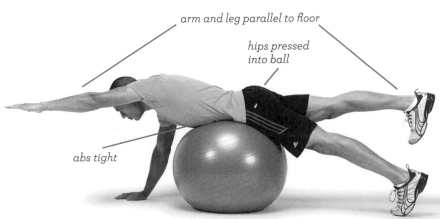

arm and leg parallel to floor

hips pressed into ball

abs tight

Position 2

> **GET MOVING**

1. As you exhale, press your hips firmly into the ball and raise your left arm to shoulder level. Extend your arm in front of you as far as you can. Simultaneously tighten your buttocks and lift your right leg, extending it as far as you can with the goal of bringing it even with your upper body. Maintain your balance with your abdominal muscles as well as your stable arm and leg. Keep your head aligned with your body. (**Position 2**) Hold this position for 2 to 5 seconds, then slowly lower your arm and leg back down to the starting position.

2. Switch sides and repeat the motion. Continue lifting opposite arms and legs as many times as you can for up to 1 minute.

TAKE 10 TIPS

Perform the Ball Balance slowly and under control. To get the most out of this exercise, keep your extended arm and leg as straight as you can.

Too hard? Tone it down
- Practice this movement without a stability ball, then add the ball when you're ready.
- Perform this movement on your hands and knees, leaning over the stability ball, raising one arm and extending the opposite leg.
- Hold this position for a shorter period of time.
- Take a break between arm/leg lifts.

Too easy? Kick it up
- Hold your arm and leg up for longer than 5 seconds.
- Perform this exercise for longer than 1 minute.

1 minute | Stretching and Deep Breathing

Ball Side Bend

EQUIPMENT: **Stability ball**
MUSCLES WORKED: **Upper and lower back, abs and waist**

I love this stretch! It's so easy that you can do it when you're relaxing at home in front of the TV. Your back will thank you.

> **GET STARTED**

Kneel down with the stability ball beside your right hip and thigh. Next, press into the ball with your right hip and side. Reach your right arm over the ball to keep it from moving. (**Position 1**)

> **GET MOVING**

1. Keeping your shoulders relaxed and squared, bend sideways over the ball to the right and press your hip into it. Remembering to breathe deeply, bend from the waist and drape yourself over the ball as far as you comfortably can.

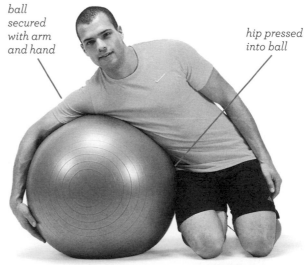

ball secured with arm and hand

hip pressed into ball

Position 1

LEVEL II

157

Place your left arm overhead and reach to the opposite side. Move your head in alignment with your upper torso. (**Position 2**) Stretch to mild tension and hold this position for up to 15 seconds.

2. Switch sides and hold for another 15 seconds.

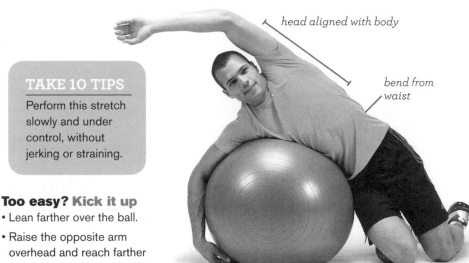

head aligned with body

bend from waist

Position 2

TAKE 10 TIPS

Perform this stretch slowly and under control, without jerking or straining.

Too hard? Tone it down
- Don't try to lean so far. Begin by leaning just a little bit and increasing inch by inch over time.
- Hold this stretch for a shorter period of time.

Too easy? Kick it up
- Lean farther over the ball.
- Raise the opposite arm overhead and reach farther as you lean to the side.
- Hold this stretch for a longer period of time.

Ball Thigh Stretch

EQUIPMENT: **Stability ball**

MUSCLES WORKED: **Fronts of legs (quads) and hips**

In sports you'll often hear a coach say, "Take a knee." This signals all the players to kneel down on one knee, usually during a time when the coach needs to talk to them. Well, I'd like you to "take a knee" because I want to tell you how proud I am of you for reaching the end of this workout. While I'm at it, I'd also like to show you the last stretch in this workout using the stability ball. If you've already been through Level I, you'll remember doing this movement with a chair (see page 112), but the stability ball takes this stretch to the next level.

> **GET STARTED** ....

Sit on top of the stability ball with your knees bent at a 90° angle. Place your feet firmly on the floor, more than shoulder-width apart. Next, slide your buttocks to the left side of the ball, with your hands on your right thigh.

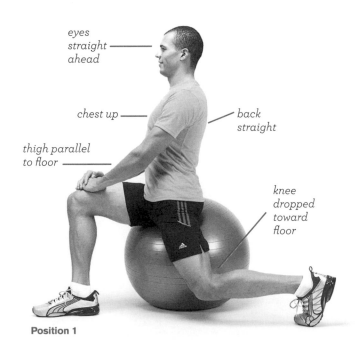

eyes straight ahead

chest up

back straight

thigh parallel to floor

knee dropped toward floor

Position 1

LEVEL II

Look straight ahead, and sit up tall and strong with your back straight. Slowly "take a knee," or drop your left knee toward the floor, while keeping the right side of your butt and right thigh on top of the ball. (**Position 1**)

▶ GET MOVING

1. With your hands still on your thigh, bend your right knee slightly and roll the ball forward, stretching your hip and the front of your left leg to the point you feel the stretch being effective. The top of your left foot will now be touching the floor. (**Position 2**) Hold this position for up to 15 seconds.

2. Now switch knees and hold the stretch on the other side for an additional 15 seconds. Remember to breathe deeply.

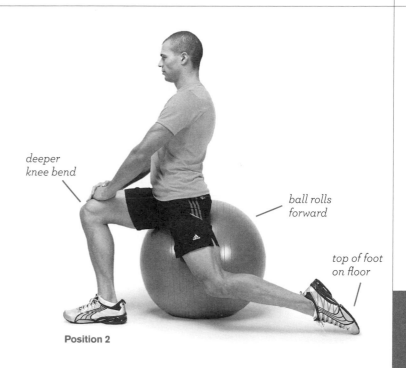

deeper knee bend

ball rolls forward

top of foot on floor

Position 2

LEVEL II

Too hard? Tone it down
- Don't roll the ball as far, and decrease the distance of your stretch.
- Hold the stretch for a shorter period of time.

Too easy? Kick it up
- Roll the ball farther forward to increase the stretch.
- Press your hip farther forward.
- Raise your arms over your head, leaning back slightly. Llongate your body by imagining yourself making a "touchdown" signal with both arms fully extended.
- Hold the stretch for a longer period of time.

TAKE 10 TIPS

Perform this stretch slowly and under control, without jerking or straining. Remember to sit up straight for the entire stretch.

You did it! Fantastic!
You have just completed your second 4•3•2•1 workout at Level II, using a resistance band and a stability ball. Now you can reward yourself or, if you prefer, go back and repeat parts of this workout or the entire circuit.

WORKOUT 3

Congratulations! You are now ready for your third workout at Level II. For this workout, you'll be using a resistance band as well as one of my all-time favorite pieces of fitness equipment: a jump rope. Jumping rope provides a great aerobic workout anywhere you'd like. Don't worry if you haven't jumped rope since first grade; I'll be showing you some tried-and-true fitness tricks to keep you from missing a step.

④ minutes | High-Energy Aerobic Training

Jumping Rope/ Jogging in Place

EQUIPMENT: Jump rope
MUSCLES WORKED: Heart, shoulders, arms, core and legs

Let me take you back to a time when moving your body was fun. Do you remember being outside in the schoolyard at recess, listening to the rhythm of whatever timeless rhymes your neighborhood used for jumping rope? I remember the girls chanting "Miss Mary Mack, Mack, Mack, all dressed in black, black, black . . ." Whatever your personal experience with the jump rope may be, I'd like to show you how a simple rope can be turned into one of the most effective fitness tools you have in your 4•3•2•1 toolbox. Jumping rope is a fantastic aerobic activity, helping you to increase your metabolism and burn body fat while toning and strengthening your muscles. Best of all, it's fun! (Note: This exercise uses the regular style of jumping rope that allows you to do an extra little hop between jumps over the rope. It does not call for the superfast jumping you may have seen boxers use as they train.)

▶ GET STARTED

Stand up straight, feet in a natural position. Hold a jump rope handle in each hand, with your shoulders relaxed and the rope behind your feet. (**Position 1**)

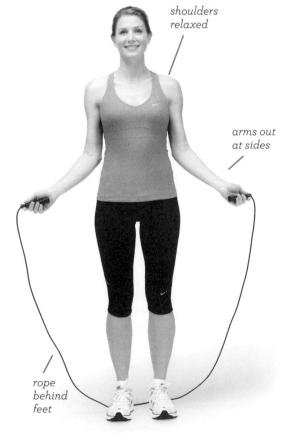

shoulders relaxed

arms out at sides

rope behind feet

Position 1

LEVEL II

160

▶ GET MOVING

1. Begin jumping rope at a moderate pace. Keeping your hands out from your body near waist level, rotate your wrists in a circular motion to move the jump rope first over your head and then under your feet. Jump over the rope by pushing off the balls of your feet. Stand tall, keeping your chest up and your shoulders relaxed. Continue jumping rope at a leisurely pace for up for 30 seconds. (**Position 2**)

2. After 30 seconds of jumping rope, stop momentarily and place the rope handles in one hand. Next, begin moderately jogging in place by raising your right knee up toward your chest with your left arm driving up toward your left shoulder, and vice versa with the other side. Keep jogging in place at a leisurely pace for 30 seconds.

3. Now it's time to jump rope again, but this time go a little faster. Keep jumping at a moderate clip for another 30 seconds. Remember, the first couple of minutes of your H.E.A.T. should be used to warm up your body, so ease into your workout, increasing your pace as you progress throughout the 4 minutes.

4. Now jog in place for 30 seconds, and then it's time to jump rope again—but this time go faster, moving your hands and feet as fast as you can, jumping rope for another 30 seconds.

5. Keep alternating Jumping Rope with Jogging in Place every 30 seconds for a total of 4 minutes. See if your "slow" jogging periods can progressively become a little faster and your "fast" jumping rope periods can get quite a bit faster.

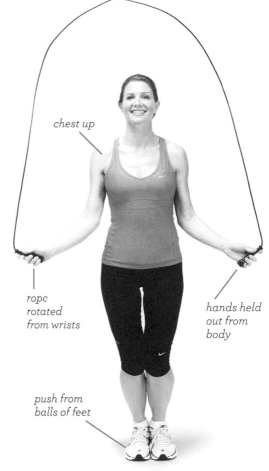

chest up

rope rotated from wrists

hands held out from body

push from balls of feet

Position 2

LEVEL II

Too hard? Tone it down

- Start with "ghost jumping." Jump up and down as if you were jumping rope but without a rope. You still get the benefit of the exercise but without the risk of tripping. Soon you may decide you want to do the real thing.

- Place both rope handles in your right hand, with the rope at the right side of your body. As you jump, rotate your right hand, moving the rope around in circles by your side. This is a great trick to help you utilize the rope as a cadence without letting it go under your feet.

- Jump slower.

- Don't jump as high.

- During the 30-second periods of moderate activity, march in place instead of jogging in place.

Too easy? Kick it up

- Move your feet and arms faster throughout the exercise.

- Jump higher.

- Jump from side to side.

- Jump on one foot.

- Perform this movement for a longer period of time.

- Alternate "fast" jumping rope (like a boxer in training, with no hop in between) with "regular" jumping rope.

TAKE 10 TIPS

To get the most out of this exercise, remember to jump from the balls of your feet and to rotate the jump rope with your wrists (not your arms). I highly recommend wearing sneakers for this exercise, not only to provide support for your feet, but also because it hurts when the rope hits your tootsies!

③ minutes | Resistance Exercise

Band Squat with Shoulder Press

EQUIPMENT: **Resistance band**

MUSCLES WORKED: **Legs, butt, shoulders and core**

Keeping in line with my approach to "fast fitness," or obtaining maximum results in minimum time, the Band Squat with Shoulder Press incorporates two movements in one exercise. Now you're multitasking!

▶ GET STARTED

Holding your resistance band with a handle in each hand, palms facing your thighs, place the middle of the band on the floor. Place both feet on top of the band, shoulder-width apart, toes slightly pointed out and knees slightly bent. Looking straight ahead and slightly up, rotate your hands so your palms are facing away from you and lift the handles up toward the front of your shoulders (this movement is like a biceps curl). Your hands should now be next to the front of your shoulders, shoulder-width apart. Rotate your hands again to position your palms facing one another (thumbs near your shoulders). Stand up straight, but relax your shoulders. (**Position 1**)

▶ GET MOVING

1. Holding the resistance band with your palms facing each other, tighten your abdominal muscles and sit back into a squat position by slowly lowering your weight down as if you were going to sit in a chair. Remember that when you're in the squat position, you should be able to draw an imaginary vertical line from your knee to the middle of your foot. Looking straight ahead and slightly up, with your head in alignment with your torso, keep your chest up and your hands at shoulder level. Go down as low as you comfortably can. (**Position 2**)

2. Next, tighten the muscles of your buttocks and push up to a standing position, pressing from your heels. Once you're in the standing position, rotate your hands, positioning them with your palms facing away from you. Next, extend both arms over your head.

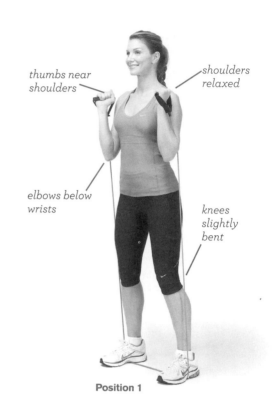

thumbs near shoulders

shoulders relaxed

elbows below wrists

knees slightly bent

Position 1

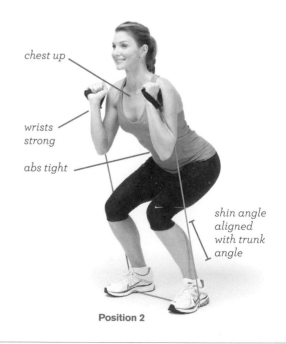

chest up

wrists strong

abs tight

shin angle aligned with trunk angle

Position 2

This is the shoulder press part of the exercise. Your torso should be tall and straight, but keep your knees and elbows slightly bent. (**Position 3**) Hold this position for 2 seconds, then slowly lower your hands back down to shoulder level.

3. Perform these two movements as many times as you can for up to 1 minute.

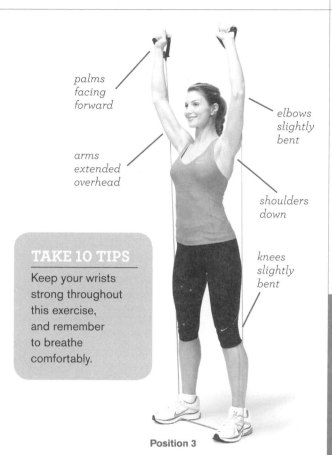

palms facing forward

elbows slightly bent

arms extended overhead

shoulders down

knees slightly bent

Position 3

Too hard? Tone it down
- Start with a quarter-squat.
- Choose a lower-level resistance band.
- Perform this movement for less than 1 minute.
- Take a breather between squats.

Too easy? Kick it up
- Go lower into your squat.
- Hold the squat position for a longer period of time.
- Raise one arm at a time when performing the shoulder press.
- Choose a higher-level resistance band.
- Perform this movement for more than 1 minute.

TAKE 10 TIPS

Keep your wrists strong throughout this exercise, and remember to breathe comfortably.

Standing Band Balance Row

EQUIPMENT: Resistance band and fixed object (door handle using door attachment or with door closed, or smooth pole, post or tree)
MUSCLES WORKED: Upper and lower back, shoulders, arms, core

This exercise incorporates two movements: balancing on one leg and moving your arms in a rowing motion. It engages a number of different muscle groups, and it's an excellent way to enhance your coordination and balance.

▶ GET STARTED

Find a fixed object to wrap your resistance band around. Loop the band around the object at waist to chest level and walk backward 2 to 3 feet, holding a handle in each hand. With your feet shoulder-width apart, bend your knees and lean back slightly. With your arms extended and elbows slightly bent, position your hands with your palms facing each other, shoulder-width apart, below chest level. (**Position 1**)

LEVEL II

Next, tighten your abdominal muscles and lift your right foot off the ground, raising it to a level that's comfortable for you. (**Position 2**)

▶ GET MOVING

1. Looking straight ahead with your head in alignment with your body, relax your shoulders and bend your elbows. As you exhale, pull both resistance band handles back toward your hips while still balancing your body on one leg. Be sure to keep your chest elevated and pull your shoulder blades together. This will enhance the training of your upper back muscles. Hold this position for 2 seconds. (**Position 3**) Then inhale and slowly extend your arms back to your starting position.

2. Perform the pulling motion with your arms as many times as you can for up to 30 seconds. Then switch legs and perform the exercise for another 30 seconds.

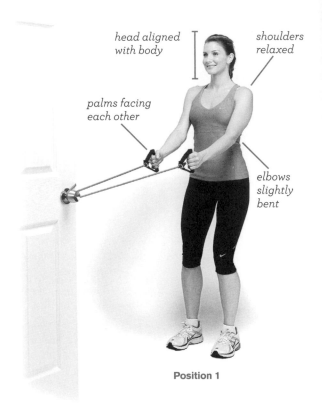

head aligned with body

shoulders relaxed

palms facing each other

elbows slightly bent

Position 1

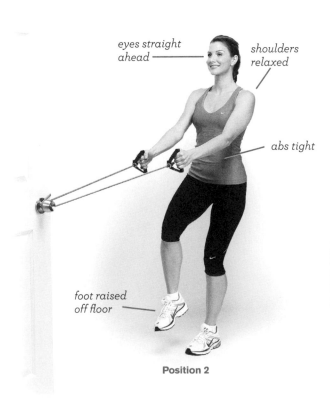

eyes straight ahead

shoulders relaxed

abs tight

foot raised off floor

Position 2

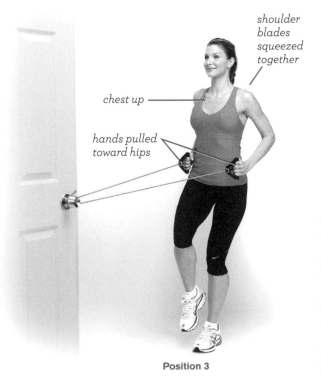

shoulder blades squeezed together

chest up

hands pulled toward hips

Position 3

Too hard? Tone it down
- Move closer to the fixed object to reduce tension on the resistance band.
- Do not attempt to bring the handles of the resistance band all the way back to your hips. You can bend your elbows slightly and then gradually increase the pull as you become stronger.
- Use a lower-level resistance band.
- Take a rest between repetitions.

Too easy? Kick it up
- Step farther away from the fixed object to increase the tension on the band.
- Raise your foot higher off the ground. Bring your knee to waist/chest level and hold for 30 seconds.
- Choose a higher-level resistance band.
- Perform the motion for longer than 1 minute.

Band Reverse Lunge with Shoulder Raise

EQUIPMENT: **Resistance band**

MUSCLES WORKED: **Legs, butt, core and shoulders**

Again, this exercise takes advantage of fitness fusion, or combining several movements into one exercise, helping you to get fit faster. When you challenge multiple muscle groups in one exercise, you not only save time but also challenge your body by recruiting muscles that you may use very little. This particular exercise is quick and simple, and can be done anywhere.

▶ GET STARTED

Holding your resistance band with a handle in each hand, place the middle of the band on the floor, then step firmly with your right foot on top of the band. (Your left foot will move back in just a moment.) Still holding the handles in each hand, position your hands and arms at your sides with your fists closed and fingers near your outer thighs. Stand tall and look straight ahead with your chest up and shoulders relaxed. (**Position 1**)

▶ GET MOVING

1. Tighten your abdominal muscles and step backward with your left foot 3 to 4 feet. Balance your weight between the heel of your right foot in front and the ball of your left foot in back. (**Position 2**)

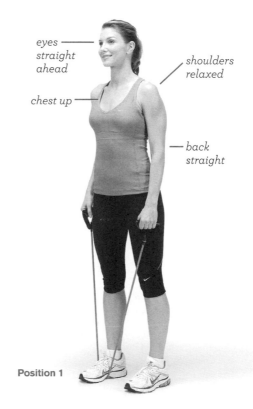

eyes straight ahead

shoulders relaxed

chest up

back straight

Position 1

LEVEL II

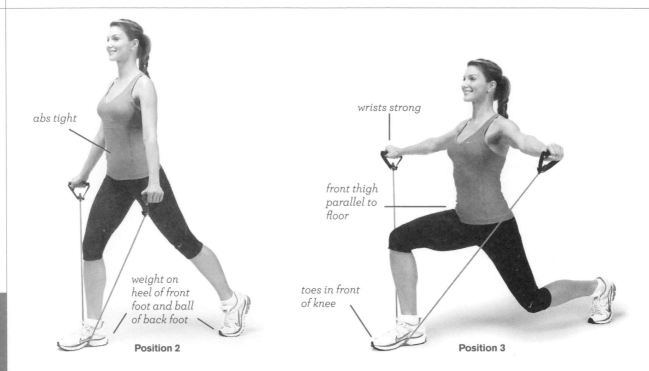

abs tight

weight on heel of front foot and ball of back foot

Position 2

wrists strong

front thigh parallel to floor

toes in front of knee

Position 3

Keeping your back straight, lower your right thigh until it's parallel to the floor (or as low as you can manage) and lower your left knee toward the floor without actually touching it. You should be able to draw an imaginary vertical line from your right knee to the middle of your right foot. Simultaneously, raise the handles of the resistance band to shoulder level (or as high as you can comfortably manage), extending your arms out and up to the side as if you were flying. (**Position 3**)

2. Next, pressing from the heel of your right foot in front and the ball of your left foot in back, push up into a standing position, while at the same time lowering the handles back down to your outer thighs. Keep your chin parallel to the floor and stay in the split-lunge position, getting ready for the next repetition.

3. Perform as many lunges and shoulder raises as you can in 30 seconds, then switch legs for an additional 30 seconds.

Too hard? Tone it down
- Rest between repetitions.
- Start with a quarter-lunge, bending your front and back legs slightly.
- Choose a lower-level resistance band.
- Perform this exercise for a shorter time frame (for example, 15 seconds for each leg).

Too easy? Kick it up
- The lower you bend your front and back legs, the more challenging this exercise will be.
- As you lower down into your lunge, raise the handles in front of your body up to shoulder level or as high as you can. Pause and then return to the starting position.
- Choose a higher-level resistance band.
- Perform the motion for longer than 1 minute.

TAKE 10 TIPS
Keep looking straight ahead—looking down at your feet can impact your balance. Remember to move at a slow and controlled pace and to keep your wrists firm and strong throughout the exercise.

② minutes | Core-Strengthening Exercises

Band Reverse Wood Chop

EQUIPMENT: Resistance band and fixed object (door handle using door attachment or with door closed, or smooth pole, post or tree)

MUSCLES WORKED: Waist, abs, back and shoulders

This exercise is related to the Band Wood Chop (see page 143), but this time you'll be pulling the resistance band away from the floor up toward your upper shoulder and ear. This exercise will help you firm up your stomach and waist.

▶ GET STARTED

Find a fixed object to wrap your resistance band around. Loop the band around the object at waist level or lower. Take a handle in each hand and step 2 to 4 feet toward the left at a diagonal, creating tension on the resistance band. Next, place your feet wider than shoulder-width apart, knees slightly bent. Extend your arms, elbows slightly bent, holding both handles to the side at waist level. Stand tall with your back straight. (**Position 1**)

▶ GET MOVING

1. Rotate your shoulders and hips away from the fixed object. While your left foot is pointing forward, you will pivot on the ball of your right foot (the one closest to the fixed object) with your heel raised. Draw your arms across the front of your body from waist to shoulder, up toward the opposite ear. Leading with your left shoulder, continue to rotate until your torso is completely turned and your hands are on the opposite side of your body. Remember to move your head with your torso. Hold this position for 2 seconds. (**Position 2**)

2. Slowly rotate your torso back to the original starting position, lowering your hands to waist level.

3. Perform as many rotations as you can to the left in 30 seconds.

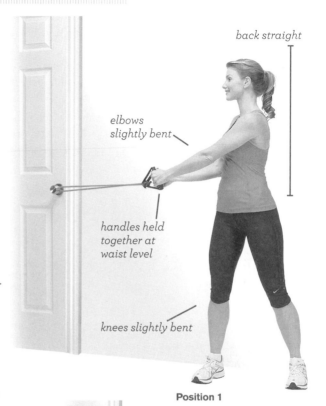

back straight

elbows slightly bent

handles held together at waist level

knees slightly bent

Position 1

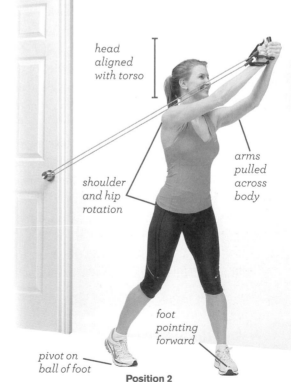

head aligned with torso

arms pulled across body

shoulder and hip rotation

foot pointing forward

pivot on ball of foot

Position 2

LEVEL II

167

4. Now reposition yourself by turning around. This time you will be holding your hands on your left, pivoting on the ball of your left foot and rotating your torso toward the right. Complete as many rotations as you can in this direction for another 30 seconds.

Too hard? Tone it down

- Step closer to the fixed object, decreasing the tension of the resistance band.
- Keep your arms bent throughout the entire motion.
- Choose a lower-level resistance band.
- Perform the movement for less than 1 minute.

Too easy? Kick it up

- Step farther to the side of the fixed object.
- Move quickly and explosively when rotating away from the fixed object, but return to your starting position slowly.
- Choose a higher-level resistance band.
- Perform the movement longer than 1 minute.

> **TAKE 10 TIPS**
>
> As you rotate your torso, allow your waist (oblique) muscles to initiate the movement as opposed to swinging your arms.

Reverse Crunch

EQUIPMENT: None (Optional: exercise mat)
MUSCLES WORKED: Core

This exercise is one of the best movements to help tone and strengthen your abdominal muscles. It's simple but effective, and you'll soon notice the benefits.

❯ GET STARTED

Begin the exercise by lying on your back, flat on the floor. Place your arms at your sides, palms on the floor, and relax your shoulders. Next, raise your knees toward your chest until they're bent at a 90° angle. Cross your ankles and bring your knees close together. This is your starting position. (**Position 1**)

❯ GET MOVING

1. While keeping your knees bent, tighten your abdominal muscles and raise your knees up toward your chest, lifting your buttocks off the floor. It's okay to press down with your palms. Imagine you're lifting your feet up toward the ceiling. Keep your head and upper back flat on the floor. Hold the highest position for 2 seconds. (**Position 2**)

2. Slowly lower your legs and feet back to your starting position.

3. Perform this movement as many times as you can in 1 minute.

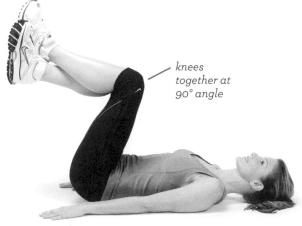

knees together at 90° angle

hands below waist, palms down

Position 1

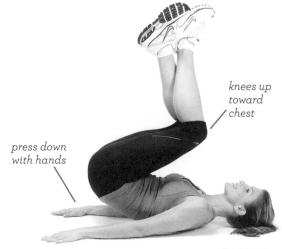

knees up toward chest

press down with hands

Position 2

Too hard? Tone it down

- Don't raise your buttocks and legs as high.
- Hold the highest position for a shorter period of time.
- Perform this exercise for a shorter period of time.

Too easy? Kick it up

- Place your hands behind your head with your elbows on the floor

throughout the motion. Do not lace your fingers behind your head.

- Straighten your legs throughout the motion and lift your legs straight up (feet to the ceiling).
- Raise your buttocks and legs higher.
- Hold the upward position longer than 2 seconds.
- Perform this exercise for longer than 1 minute.

TAKE 10 TIPS

It's very important to control the descent when lowering your legs back to the starting position (keep it slow), as this part of the exercise will also give your abs a great workout.

1 minute | Stretching and Deep Breathing

Lying Spinal Twist

EQUIPMENT: **None**

MUSCLES WORKED: **Lower back and hips**

This is a great stretch for a tight or tired lower back. You can do this exercise when you're lying down, relaxing to some soothing music, or when you're just about to hit the sack. It's easy to perform, and I promise you'll like the results.

❯ GET STARTED

Lie on your back on the floor with your legs extended and your feet together. Place your hands, palms facing down, on the floor out to the side at shoulder level. Keeping your shoulders on the floor, put your right foot next to your left knee. (**Position 1**)

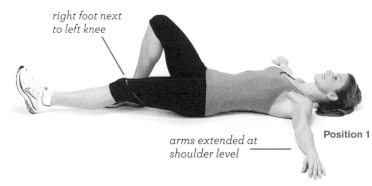

right foot next to left knee

arms extended at shoulder level

Position 1

❯ GET MOVING

1. Next, place your left hand on the side of your right knee and gently pull the right knee down toward the floor. Gently stretch your lower back while keeping your right shoulder and arm pressed to the floor. Also, look in the opposite direction as your hips are turning—that is, toward your right hand and shoulder. (**Position 2**)

2. Hold this position for as long as you comfortably can—up to 15 seconds—then switch sides for another 15 seconds.

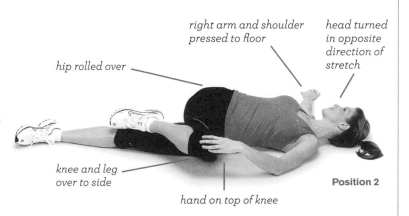

right arm and shoulder pressed to floor

head turned in opposite direction of stretch

hip rolled over

knee and leg over to side

hand on top of knee

Position 2

LEVEL II

Too hard? Tone it down
• Don't roll your hips over as far.
• Hold this stretch for a shorter period of time.

Too easy? Kick it up
• Raise the knee you are stretching nearer your shoulder.
• Straighten your top leg as you roll your hips to the side.
• Hold the stretch for a longer period of time.

Shoulder Back Stretch

EQUIPMENT: None (Optional: exercise mat)
MUSCLES WORKED: Upper and lower back and shoulders

Here's your last stretch for this workout—I saved the best for last! I call this the stretch of "royalty"! This exercise is not unlike a loyal subject prostrating himself on the floor before his honored queen or king. This is a great, simple stretch to rejuvenate your upper and lower back as well as your shoulders. I especially like to perform this exercise before bed to help calm and relax my body and mind.

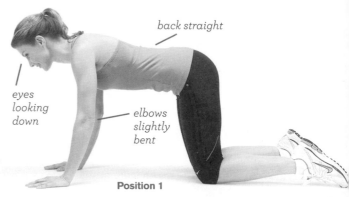

back straight

eyes looking down

elbows slightly bent

Position 1

▶ GET STARTED

Begin this movement by positioning your body on all fours, hands and knees on the floor, with your back straight. Keeping your head in alignment with your body, look down and keep your elbows slightly bent. (**Position 1**)

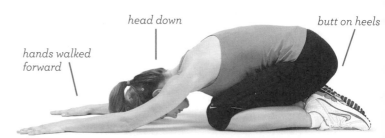

head down

butt on heels

hands walked forward

Position 2

▶ GET MOVING

1. Sit back, shifting your butt back on your heels while lowering down on your forearms. Bending from the waist, walk your hands forward, allowing your head to drop between your shoulders. (**Position 2**)

2. Hold this stretch as long as you can, up to 30 seconds.

Too hard? Tone it down
• Decrease the distance of your stretch.
• Hold the stretch for a shorter period of time.

Too easy? Kick it up
• Increase the distance of your stretch.
• Hold the stretch for a longer period of time.

Well done!
You have just completed your third 4•3•2•1 workout at Level II!
Now you can give yourself a reward—or, if you're so inclined,
go back and repeat parts of the workout or the entire circuit.

LEVEL II

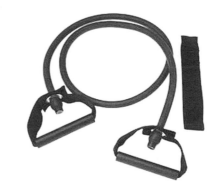

WORKOUT 4

This fourth workout combines everything you've learned in the first three workouts and then some! Now I'm going to "raise the bar"—or should I say "raise the band"? In this workout, you'll learn a brand-new H.E.A.T. technique, more advanced resistance training exercises and a more challenging core routine—all using the exercise band! What are we waiting for . . . let's strike up the band!

④ minutes | High-Energy Aerobic Training

Hopscotch Shuffle

EQUIPMENT: Resistance bands
MUSCLES WORKED: Heart, core and legs

Did you ever hopscotch as a kid? For many of us, moving our bodies used to be as natural as breathing. In fact, if we didn't have time to run around, we felt crabby, irritable and bored. Much of the development of my 4•3•2•1 program came from watching children play and then figuring out how to help adults get fit while they reexperienced the joys of childhood games. I'd like to take you back to another childhood experience, this time performing two movements that together create a powerful H.E.A.T. experience. This fantastic aerobic activity improves your coordination and agility, burns calories, increases your metabolism, burns body fat, and tones and strengthens your muscles. It's a lot of fun, too. Ready to play?

▶ GET STARTED

Make a "+" on the floor by laying a resistance band down horizontally (east to west) and crossing it with another resistance band (or jump rope) vertically (north to south). If you prefer, you can use chalk to make the mark on the ground or sidewalk. You'll be coming back to this later.

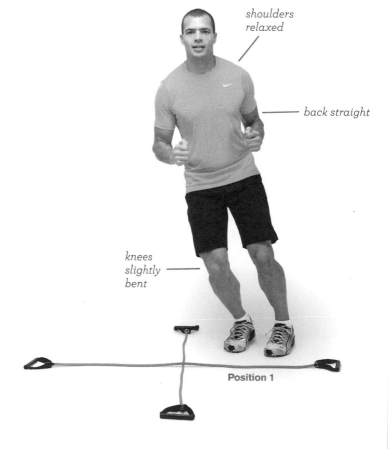

shoulders relaxed

back straight

knees slightly bent

Position 1

▶ GET MOVING

1. Begin this exercise by jogging in place to warm up your muscles. Raise your right knee up toward your chest and your left arm toward your shoulder. Keep your back straight and bring your hands all the way from your hips to your shoulders. After 30 seconds of jogging in place, stop and stand in one of the quadrants made by the band.

2. Start with both feet together and knees slightly bent. (**Position 1**) Jump to the other side of the band by pushing off the balls of your feet. (**Position 2**) Quickly jump back to the first side. Continue this motion as fast as you can, jumping from side to side over the band. You will naturally lean forward slightly from the waist as you jump, so focus on keeping your chest up, your back straight, your shoulders relaxed and your head in alignment with your torso. Also, while keeping your arms basically at a 90° angle with your hands comfortably in front of your body (imagine you're holding a ski pole in each hand and you're a mogul skier racing in the Olympics), allow your hands and arms to move naturally from side to side as you jump back and forth. Jump as fast as you comfortably can for 30 seconds.

3. Keep alternating 30 seconds of moderate jogging in place with 30 seconds of intense Hopscotch Shuffle, for a total of 4 minutes. See if your jogging periods can progressively become a little faster and your jumping can get quite a bit faster.

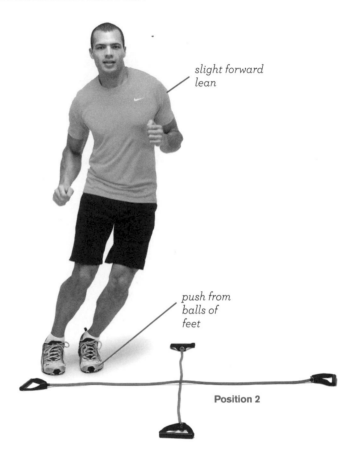

slight forward lean

push from balls of feet

Position 2

Too hard? Tone it down
- Instead of jogging in place, try Marching in Place (see page 123).
- Jump over the band more slowly.
- Don't jump over the band as high.
- Keep your hands on your hips throughout the movement.

Too easy? Kick it up
- Move your feet and arms more quickly as you jog.
- Jump faster.
- Jump higher.
- Jump on one foot.
- Hold your arms out to the sides at shoulder level as you jump.
- Mix it up by jumping between quadrants—side to side, up and back, even diagonally.
- Perform this movement for a longer period of time.

TAKE 10 TIPS

To get the most out of this exercise, remember to jump using the balls of your feet. Think of being "light" on your feet as you jump back and forth or from side to side.

LEVEL II

③ minutes | Resistance Exercise

Band Overhead Squat

EQUIPMENT: Resistance band
MUSCLES WORKED: Shoulders, core, butt and legs

This exercise is deceptive. It looks simple, but when you perform it, you will know it's providing a significant challenge to your entire body. You'll be performing a squat motion while holding the handles of your resistance band above your head—yes, throughout the entire exercise! This variation provides a great workout for your core, making your abs and lower back work overtime. After attempting this movement, you'll probably agree that *one* minute can be a workout!

▶ GET STARTED

Holding your resistance band with a handle in each hand, place the middle of the band on the floor and then step on top of the band with both feet, placing them shoulder-width apart with your toes pointed slightly out. Looking ahead and slightly up, rotate your hands so your palms are facing you and lift the handles up to shoulder level (this movement is like a biceps curl). Next, rotate your hands so your palms are facing each other. (**Position 1**)

▶ GET MOVING

1. Next, rotate your hands so your palms are facing forward. Extend both arms up, pressing the resistance band handles over your head. Imagine that someone is pointing a gun at you and saying, "Stick 'em up—and reach for the sky!" Make sure both arms are extended, with elbows slightly bent. Still looking straight ahead, keep your chest up, tighten your abdominal muscles and sit back into a squat position, slowly lowering your weight down as if you were going to sit in a chair. As with all other squat motions, be sure your knees don't extend over your toes when you're in the squat position. Also, keep your head in alignment with your torso. Keep holding your resistance band handles above your head. The goal of this movement is to keep your hands and arms as far back as you can as you lower down into the squat position, so push your arms and shoulders back. Go down as low as you comfortably can. (**Position 2**)

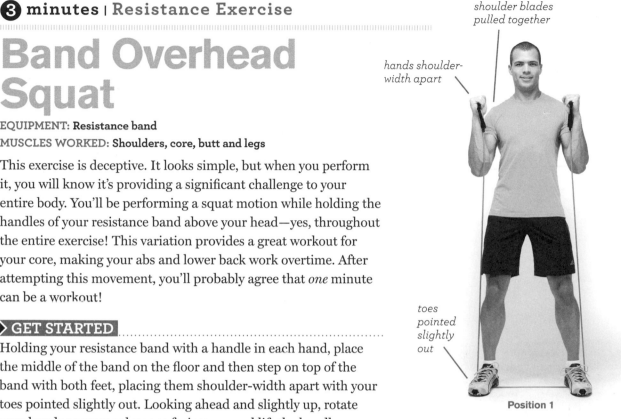

shoulder blades
pulled together

hands shoulder-
width apart

toes
pointed
slightly
out

Position 1

LEVEL II

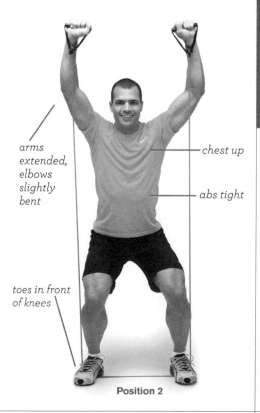

arms
extended,
elbows
slightly
bent

chest up

abs tight

toes in front
of knees

Position 2

173

2. Next, tighten the muscles of your buttocks and push up to a standing position by pressing from your heels—all the while keeping your arms extended over your head with your elbows slightly bent.

3. Perform as many squats as you can in 1 minute.

Too hard? Tone it down
- Start with a quarter-squat.
- Choose a lower-level resistance band.
- When you stand up, bring your arms down and rest.
- Perform this movement for less than 1 minute.
- Take a breather between squats.

Too easy? Kick it up
- Go lower into your squat.
- Hold the squat for a longer period of time.
- Choose a higher-level resistance band.
- Perform this movement for more than 1 minute.

TAKE 10 TIPS

Remember to keep your wrists firm and strong throughout this exercise. Also, to help your balance, hold your arms wider than shoulder-width apart and keep your chest up while looking straight ahead.

Lunge with Band Balance Row

EQUIPMENT: **Resistance band and fixed object (door handle using door attachment or with door closed, or smooth pole, post or tree)**

MUSCLES WORKED: **Upper and lower back, butt, legs, core, shoulders and arms**

Here's some more 4•3•2•1 math: How would you like to train more than seven different muscle groups while performing just two simple movements in one exercise? This challenging exercise does just that, strengthening your entire body while enhancing your coordination and balance. Using the resistance band, you are going to incorporate a lower body movement (the Stationary Lunge) with an upper body movement (the Band Balance Row) in a fitness fusion format. You'll also feel your heart rate quicken, which is key for getting that metabolic boost.

> **GET STARTED** ....

Find a fixed object to wrap your resistance band around. Loop the band around the object at waist level or lower. Next, with a handle in each hand, walk backward (facing the fixed object) 1 to 3 feet, keeping your arms extended, to increase the tension on the band. Now step backward 2 to 3 feet with your left foot and assume the split-stance position.

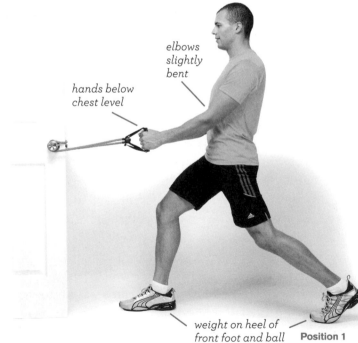

elbows slightly bent

hands below chest level

weight on heel of front foot and ball of back foot

Position 1

Balance your weight between the heel of your right foot in front and the ball of your left foot in back. Hold a band handle in each hand, with your palms facing each other and both arms extended, elbows slightly bent. Your hands should be below chest level. (**Position 1**)

❯ GET MOVING

1. Keeping your chest up, your chin parallel to the floor and your back straight, tighten your abdominal muscles and pull both resistance band handles back toward your hips. Draw your elbows back as far as possible. Think of squeezing your shoulder blades together. This will enhance the training of your upper back muscles. At the same time, lower yourself into a lunge position. Your right thigh should be parallel to the floor (or as low as you can manage), and your left knee should dip down toward the floor without touching it. You should be able to draw an imaginary vertical line from your front knee to the middle of your foot. Balance your weight between the heel of your right foot in front and the ball of your left foot in back and hold this position for 2 seconds. (**Position 2**)

2. Next, extend your arms back to the starting position while maintaining a stationary lunge.

3. Perform as many repetitions as you can in 30 seconds. Then switch legs and continue for another 30 seconds.

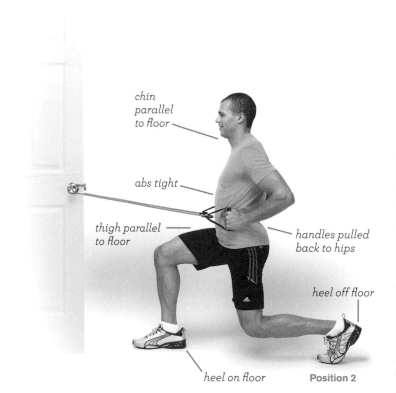

chin parallel to floor

abs tight

thigh parallel to floor

handles pulled back to hips

heel off floor

heel on floor

Position 2

Too hard? Tone it down

- Move closer to the fixed object to reduce the tension on the resistance band.
- Do a quarter-lunge instead of a full lunge.
- Do not pull the handles of the resistance band all the way back.
- Choose a lower-level resistance band.
- Take a rest between repetitions.

Too easy? Kick it up

- Step farther away from the fixed object to increase the tension on the band.
- Choose a higher-level resistance band.
- Perform the motion longer than 1 minute.

TAKE 10 TIPS

Throughout this exercise, be sure your head is in alignment with your body. Keep your back straight, with your eyes looking straight ahead. Don't forget to breathe! Exhale as you pull the band handles toward your hips and inhale as you extend your arms.

Band Step-Up with Shoulder Raise

EQUIPMENT: Resistance band and bench (or steps or chair) 8 to 18 inches in height

MUSCLES WORKED: Legs, butt, core and shoulders

Are you a balanced individual? By that I mean, can you balance your body efficiently? As we get older, our coordination and balance tend to diminish. But this exercise is designed to improve your balance and coordination. Using a bench and a resistance band, it combines a shoulder exercise with a step-up motion. This is a great exercise to perform outside in a park next to a bench or on some steps.

❯ GET STARTED

Holding your resistance band with a handle in each hand, stand facing a park bench or platform (about 8 to 18 inches high) Next, place the center of the band on the bench, platform, stair or chair and step firmly with your right foot on top of the band on the bench. Make sure you don't extend your knee over your right foot when stepping up on the bench. Leave your left foot on the ground. Keeping your wrists strong, position your hands out to the sides of your body, increasing the tension on the band and helping you balance. Stand up straight, with your chin parallel to the ground. (**Position 1**)

❯ GET MOVING

1. Tighten your abdominal muscles and step up, pressing from the heel of your right foot on the bench and the ball of your left foot on the ground. Bring your left foot up on top of the bench, with your feet now firmly positioned on the bench hip-width apart. (**Position 2**) Next, raise the handles of the resistance band out to the sides of your body. Try to hold the handles at shoulder level. Hold this position for 2 seconds. (**Position 3**)

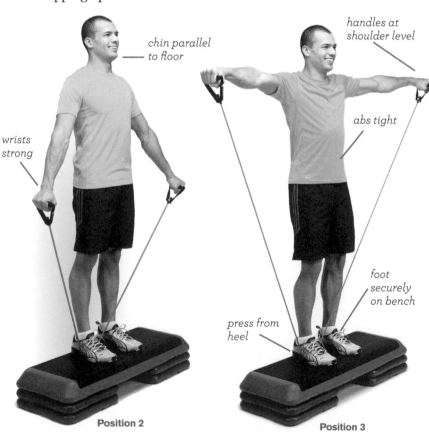

chin parallel to floor

toes in front of knee

Position 1

chin parallel to floor

wrists strong

Position 2

handles at shoulder level

abs tight

foot securely on bench

press from heel

Position 3

LEVEL II

2. Next, lower your hands down to your sides (while keeping tension on the band) and then lower your left foot back to the ground. Move at a slow and controlled pace. Leave your right foot on top of the bench with the band underneath.

3. Perform as many repetitions as you can in 30 seconds, then switch legs and complete as many repetitions as you can for an additional 30 seconds.

Too hard? Tone it down
- Select a lower bench.
- Rest between repetitions.
- Don't hold the band handles as high.
- Choose a lower-level resistance band.
- Perform this exercise for a shorter time frame (for example, 15 seconds each leg).

Too easy? Kick it up
- Select a higher bench.
- Raise the handles of the resistance band above your head in a shoulder press, as if you were making a "touchdown" signal. Lower them as you step down from the bench.
- Raise the handles of the resistance band in front of your body. Start with the handles near your thighs, with your palms facing your thighs. As you step up, raise your hands up as high as you can, with the goal of reaching shoulder level. Lower them as you step down from the bench.
- Choose a higher-level resistance band.
- Perform the exercise for longer than 1 minute.

> **TAKE 10 TIPS**
>
> As you do this exercise, imagine that you're a tightrope walker, holding your hands out to the side for balance. Maintaining tension on the resistance band during the entire exercise will help you keep your balance. Also, look straight ahead—looking down at your feet can affect your balance. Remember to breathe comfortably and to keep your wrists firm.

LEVEL II

2 minutes | Core-Strengthening Exercises

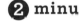

Band Pull Crunch

EQUIPMENT: Resistance band and fixed object (door handle using door attachment and with door closed, or smooth pole, post or tree limb)
MUSCLES WORKED: Core (lower back and abs)

This exercise strengthens and tones your abs and back muscles without straining your neck or lower back. I love this exercise because there are multiple ways to increase or decrease its intensity.

> GET STARTED
Find a horizontal fixed object that's high enough off the ground to provide tension on your resistance band. (If you're using a door, use a door attachment and close the door securely.) Loop the middle of the band around the object above your head. Kneel down facing the object, positioning your knees and feet hip-width apart. Hold a band handle in each hand near the sides (temples) of your head. (**Position 1**)

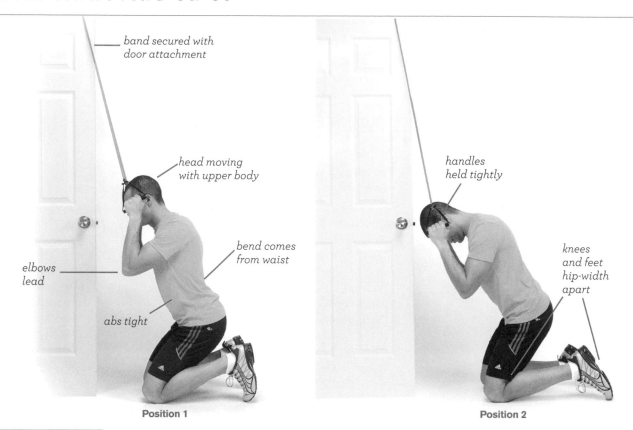

band secured with door attachment

head moving with upper body

handles held tightly

bend comes from waist

elbows lead

knees and feet hip-width apart

abs tight

Position 1

Position 2

❯ GET MOVING

1. Make sure your back is straight and your shoulders are relaxed. As you exhale, tighten your abdominal muscles and bend down from the waist, leading with your elbows. Keeping your head in alignment with your body, bring your shoulders and elbows down to the middle of your thighs. Hold the downward position for 2 seconds. (**Position 2**)

2. Moving slowly and under control, allow your body to rise up to the starting position as you inhale.

3. Perform this movement as many times as you can in 1 minute.

> ### TAKE 10 TIPS
>
> To get the most out of this exercise, move slowly on the way down and on the way back up. Also, remember to begin by contracting your abs to lean down.

Too hard? Tone it down

- Widen your base by placing your knees shoulder-width apart.
- Move closer to the fixed object, decreasing the tension on the resistance band.
- Choose a lower-level resistance band.
- Perform this exercise for less than 1 minute.
- Perform this exercise while seated in a chair. Holding the resistance band with a handle in each hand, loop the middle of the band around the back of a square-backed chair. Next, hold both handles in one hand as you sit on the edge of the chair. Place both feet on the ground with knees bent at a 90° angle shoulder-width apart. Now transfer one handle to the other hand and position the band around your shoulders and hold at chest level. Next, lean forward, bending from the waist, contracting your abs and drawing your elbows down toward your knees. Note: When performing this movement in a chair, be sure the resistance band is secure.

Too easy? Kick it up

- Place your knees and feet closer together when kneeling down.
- Position yourself farther away from the fixed object to increase the tension on the resistance band.
- Shorten the band by wrapping it one or two times around the original loop.
- Choose a higher-level resistance band.
- Perform the movement for longer than 1 minute.

Single-Leg Bridge

EQUIPMENT: None (Optional: Exercise mat)
MUSCLES WORKED: Back, core, butt and legs

The Single-Leg Bridge is a challenging core exercise that doesn't require any equipment at all—just a small space to lie down and away you go! Even though this exercise uses bodyweight, I have included it in Level II because—as you'll see—it's more difficult than the movements in Level I.

▶ GET STARTED

Begin by lying on your back with your knees bent and your feet placed firmly on the floor, hip-width apart. Place your arms by your sides with your palms facing down. (**Position 1**)

▶ GET MOVING

1. Tighten your abdominal muscles and raise your hips off the floor. (**Position 2**) Once you're in the bridge position, transfer your weight onto your left leg, then straighten your right leg and lift it off the ground. Tighten the muscles of your buttocks and press down with your upper back and shoulders, your palms and the heel of your left foot. (**Position 3**) Continue to keep your hips elevated, holding your right leg as straight as you can. Your head and shoulders should not leave the floor. Also, exhale as you raise your hips and breathe comfortably as you stay in the Single-Leg Bridge position. Hold this elevated position for 30 seconds or as long as you can.

2. Lower your hips and touch your buttocks to the floor, then immediately go right back up to complete another bridge, this time straightening the opposite leg for an additional 30 seconds.

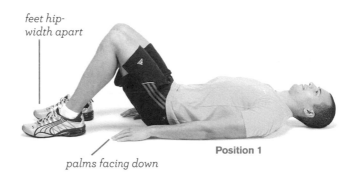

feet hip-width apart
Position 1
palms facing down

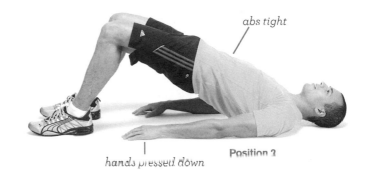

abs tight
hands pressed down
Position 2

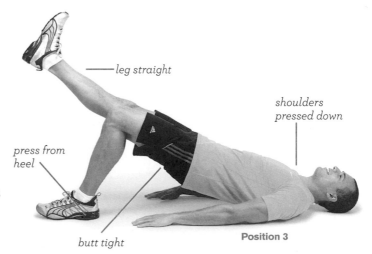

leg straight
shoulders pressed down
press from heel
butt tight
Position 3

Too hard? Tone it down

- Keep both feet on the floor and raise your hips into the bridge position.

- Lie on the floor between repetitions and take a rest.

- Hold the upward position for a shorter period of time (for example, 10 seconds for each leg instead of 30).

Too easy? Kick it up

- Hold the upward bridge position for a longer period of time.

- Perform the exercise for longer than 1 minute.

TAKE 10 TIPS

As in all core movements, remember to move slowly and under control. Also, exhale as you raise your hips—breathe comfortably as you hold the bridge position and then slowly lower down and inhale deeply.

1 minute | Stretching and Deep Breathing

Touching Toe Walk

EQUIPMENT: **None**

MUSCLES WORKED: **Upper and lower back, backs of legs and lower legs (calves and ankles)**

The next two stretching movements are called *dynamic stretching,* meaning you move your body and stretch your muscles at the same time. This kind of stretching is quite invigorating and gives you an extra boost of energy anytime you need it.

▶ GET STARTED

Stand with your feet together and knees slightly bent, holding your hands out in front of your thighs, palms down. Next, bending from the waist, begin to lower your hands down toward the floor to touch your toes. (Don't worry if you can't touch your toes—in time you'll get there!) (**Position 1**)

▶ GET MOVING

1. Lean forward and out, placing your palms on the floor and distributing your weight between your palms and the balls of your feet. Looking down, walk your hands out into a push-up position. (**Position 2**)

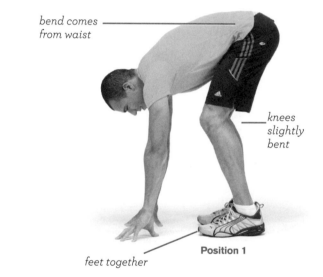

bend comes from waist

knees slightly bent

feet together

Position 1

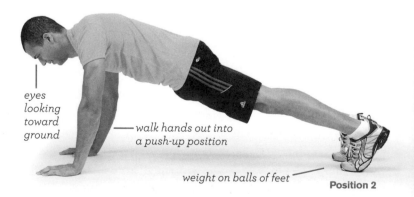

eyes looking toward ground

walk hands out into a push-up position

weight on balls of feet

Position 2

2. Keeping your hands in the same position, slowly walk your feet up toward your hands. Bend from your waist and keep your legs as straight as you can as you make small "inch by inch" toe-heel steps. Walk your feet up as far as you can. (**Position 3**) Once you arrive at a distance where you experience a stretch in the backs of your legs and lower back, shift your weight to your heels and hold the stretch for 5 seconds before walking your hands out into a push-up position and beginning the movement again.

3. Continue this exercise for 30 seconds.

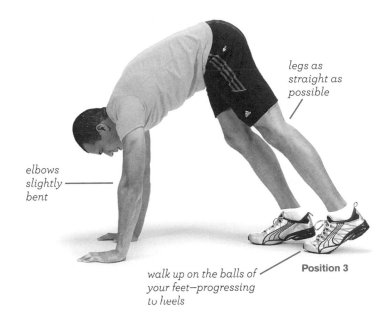

legs as straight as possible

elbows slightly bent

walk up on the balls of your feet—progressing to heels

Position 3

Too hard? Tone it down
- Decrease the distance of your stretch.
- Hold this stretch for a shorter period of time.

Too easy? Kick it up
- Increase the distance of your stretch.
- Hold the stretch for a longer period of time.

TAKE 10 TIPS

Keep your head in alignment with your body and breathe deeply throughout this stretch. Move slowly and under control, without jerking or straining.

Airplane

EQUIPMENT: **None**

MUSCLES WORKED: **Upper and lower back and backs of legs (hamstrings)**

When I was little, I would run around the house playing airplane, pretending to soar through imaginary clouds with my arms spread out as wings. If you did, too, then this stretch should be a breeze for you. Even if you didn't play airplane, you'll find this stretch makes you feel as if you could fly.

▶ GET STARTED

Stand with your back straight and your feet together, knees slightly bent and hands held out in front of your thighs, palms down.

▶ GET MOVING

1. Bend forward from the waist, as if bowing to an audience, and lower your chest until your back is parallel to the ground. At the same time, lift your left leg and extend it behind you. Tighten the muscles of your buttocks and raise your left leg as high as you comfortably can. Try to raise it to be in line with your back. The knee of your standing leg should be slightly bent.

Once you feel that you're balanced, extend both arms out to the side, as if you were an airplane. Keep your shoulders relaxed and your head in alignment with your body. (**Position 1**) Hold this position for 5 seconds.

2. Alternate legs and make an airplane as many times as you can in 30 seconds.

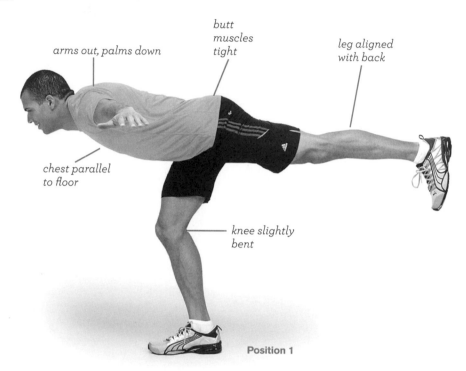

butt muscles tight

arms out, palms down

leg aligned with back

chest parallel to floor

knee slightly bent

Position 1

Too hard? Tone it down
- Decrease the distance of your stretch (not bending as far forward).
- Hold the stretch for a shorter period of time.

Too easy? Kick it up
- Increase the distance of your stretch (bending farther forward).
- Hold the stretch for a longer period of time.

TAKE 10 TIPS

Remember to move slowly and under control, without jerking or straining, and to breathe deeply throughout this stretch.

Way to go!

You have just completed the final workout in Level II. Feel free to take a break or, if you prefer, go back and repeat parts of the workout or the entire circuit. Or you can have a party and celebrate how much you've accomplished this month! Complete the assessment on page 257 to determine how much your fitness has changed in the last month. Are you ready to go on to Level III? Or do you wish to repeat Level II, only making the exercises more challenging this time? Don't worry—either decision is the right one!

chapter 9

Level III: Moving Ahead

Fitness Using Gym Equipment

By now you have mastered both Level I and Level II of the 10-Minute Total Body Breakthrough program. This is a huge accomplishment! You have been exercising every day for 10 minutes, you've learned eight 4•3•2•1 workouts and have followed the daily instructions for 56 days, and you've been making healthy eating choices and keeping your body appropriately fueled every few hours. The differences between the "old you" and the "new you" must be dramatic!

The next four workouts use three more pieces of equipment: dumbbells, a medicine ball and barbells. You can purchase these for your home gym or use them at a workout center. If you're not familiar with these items, don't be intimidated—I'll show you exactly how to use them safely and effectively. If you're already paying for a gym membership, this chapter will show you how to get even more out of it!

Why Go to a Gym?

You have completed four weeks of workouts based on your own bodyweight, and four weeks of workouts using the jump rope, stability ball and resistance bands in your home exercise area. Now you're ready for a greater challenge: going to a gym or fitness center, or adding dumbbells, a medicine ball, barbells and a bench to your home gym. In the list below, find the benefits of joining a gym that appeal to you.

- A gym has thousands of dollars worth of specialized equipment for you to test and, if you like it, use on a regular basis.

- A gym has graduated weights and resistance bands so you don't have to purchase a range of them yourself.

- A gym has the latest and greatest in cardiovascular equipment. If a treadmill with a built-in monitor is important to you, let the gym pay for it.

- Gyms and fitness centers offer additional classes if you're interested in kickboxing, Pilates, dancing, spinning or other activities.

- Some gyms and fitness centers offer multiple facilities, such as a swimming pool, track or racquetball courts.

- Many gyms provide child care.

- Most gyms have fitness experts to teach you how to perform exercises correctly and to "spot" you when you're working with heavy weights.

- Going to the gym allows you to meet other people. Exercising with others is fun and keeps you motivated.

- Some fitness centers offer bloodwork and other fitness evaluations.

- Some health clubs have extra luxuries. A spa, juice bar or fitness clothing store can make your trip that much more enjoyable.

When choosing a gym, look for one that's not too far from your home. In addition to the benefits just listed, you'll want to consider how expensive it is, how clean it is, the hours it's open, whether or not it's fully air-conditioned, and what the rules are about occasionally bringing a friend along.

Suggested Equipment for Level III

You can use the three types of exercise equipment described below at your favorite fitness center or purchase them for your home gym. Each item has its own, unique qualities to make your workouts that much more challenging, effective—and fun!

Dumbbells

One of the fastest ways to get your body lean and strong is to use dumbbells. They offer your body one of the most challenging workouts it can have. Among other benefits:

- *Dumbbells provide a free range of motion.* Unlike weight machines, dumbbells allow your body to experience movement in multiple directions. This maximizes the number of muscles affected and minimizes injuries due to the size or design of weight machines.

- *Dumbbells provide a greater variety of exercises and allow you to perform compound movements.* You can perform multiple movements in one exercise, getting more reward for your investment of time.

- *Dumbbells allow you to train one arm at a time.* If one arm is stronger than the other, dumbbells will make it obvious. When you exercise with a dumbbell using one arm, your body has no way of compensating, or allowing your stronger arm to take over.

- *Dumbbells are safer than other weight equipment.* People do occasionally drop weights, due to fatigue or mishandling. It's better to drop a dumbbell to the floor than a barbell on *you*!

- *Dumbbells recruit other muscles for balance.* As you perform dumbbell exercises, stabilizing muscles kick in to help support your body.

If you wish to purchase dumbbells for your home gym, consider your space concerns as well as your specific workout goals. If your goal is toning your body in general, I recommend purchasing two or three sets of regular dumbbells (for example, sets that are 8, 12 and 15 pounds). This allows you to perform a variety of exercises but limits the number of dumbbells underfoot in your home exercise area. If your goal is to build muscle size and strength, I recommend purchasing adjustable dumbbells, also called "stack" dumbbells. These dumbbells allow you to select the weight you need for a particular exercise with a convenient twist-and-lock system. They're more expensive than regular dumbbells, but they're perfect for people who plan to use multiple amounts of weights and don't want a roomful of 20 different-size regular dumbbells.

You can purchase different types of dumbbells at any sporting goods store, or go to www.4321fitness .com and we'll help you locate a supplier with quality products and reasonable prices.

Medicine Ball

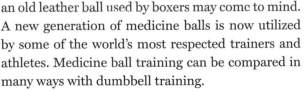

Back in the 1900s, the word "medicine" suggested health or exercise. You may remember playing with a large, heavy stuffed ball called a medicine ball when you were a kid. Visions of an old leather ball used by boxers may come to mind. A new generation of medicine balls is now utilized by some of the world's most respected trainers and athletes. Medicine ball training can be compared in many ways with dumbbell training.

- *A medicine ball provides a variety of exercises.* The versatility of training movements using a medicine ball is endless. It can be used in any plane of motion, and it allows you to toss, swing, bounce and throw. You can perform lower-body jump movements, upper-body throwing exercises and core-twisting motions. Try doing all that with a dumbbell! You can really think out of the box when it comes to training with this apparatus.

- *A medicine ball enhances athleticism.* Unlike other types of equipment, it allows you to develop hand-eye coordination, muscular strength, power, balance and endurance.

- *A medicine ball is excellent for functional exercises.* Many of the movements we perform on a daily basis involve bending, twisting and reaching. These functional movements can be strengthened with medicine ball training.

Medicine balls for your home gym are available in sizes from 1 pound to 50 pounds, and they come in all shapes, sizes, colors and prices, up to about $60. Some have handles, and some come with different accessories. I recommend starting out with a lighter medicine ball to ensure that you perform the recommended exercises correctly. You want a ball heavy enough to be challenging but not so heavy that it will limit your technique, range of motion, or safety. To determine the ideal weight, try a couple of movements using dumbbells of different weights. Not all medicine ball movements can be replicated using a dumbbell, so it's a good idea to go to your local sporting goods store to try out the real thing before you buy.

My favorite medicine balls are the ones that bounce. This allows you to perform multiple throwing and slamming movements. I recommend Xerball medicine balls from SPRI Products, as we have used these in our classes for years. Once you know what weight, color and size you want, you can purchase the ball(s) from your local sporting goods store or go to www.4321fitness.com and look for the link to our partner stores.

Barbells

You've probably seen many pictures of strong men and women performing amazing feats of strength, lifting barbells that bend with hundreds of pounds of weight. But what you might not understand is what barbell training can do for you. Consider the benefits of barbell training outlined below:

- *Barbells provide a progressive muscle challenge.* When a muscle is challenged, it responds by getting stronger. To facilitate this process, your muscles must be *progressively* challenged— that is, you must keep lifting more weight. A barbell provides the perfect opportunity to incrementally challenge your muscles as you get stronger.

- *Barbells challenge the major muscle groups.* One of the greatest benefits of barbell training is that you can perform movements that involve multiple muscle groups. These movements require great exertion and a level of weight that cannot be accomplished with dumbbells or medicine balls.

- *Barbells allow advanced power generation.* Barbells are great for performing Olympic (and non-Olympic) movements such as the snatch and the clean and jerk. These movements, for advanced individuals only, dramatically improve overall body strength.

Purchasing barbells for your home gym is a big investment. At most sporting goods stores, you can find barbells ranging from $125 to $500. You can also purchase barbell amenities such as a squat rack or a bench. I recommend trying the barbell at the store before purchasing. Make sure it's a high-quality bar, both for safety reasons and because you'll most likely be adding more weights. Go to www.4321fitness.com and look for our reputable partner stores.

If You're Starting at Level III . . .

A few fitness buffs and athletes may be fit enough to begin here at Level III. To do this, you must be familiar with the movements covered in previous workouts. If you believe you're ready for Level III, I recommend that you first perform all four workouts at the end of Level II, using the tips for making the exercises as challenging as possible. You may find that Level II is not as easy as you thought.

If you've completed the workouts in Level II at their most challenging and still are convinced that you should begin at Level III, then read the information about timing your workouts (page 90), the Intensity Scale (page 91), and warming up (page 91). I also strongly suggest that you read the 56 days of daily instructions in Chapter 10 for Level I and Level II to get the benefit of all the FUEL, RENEW and CONNECT tips.

Why No High-Tech Gym Equipment?

As a personal trainer, I often design exercise routines that use expensive, specialized, high-tech equipment that can be found only at the gym. These machines are an excellent way to get into shape, but they are not an option for most home gyms. For this reason, I have purposely kept the equipment in Level III low-tech.

More important, when you've come to the end of Level III, I want you to use the flip cards at the back of the book to mix-and-match different sections from different workouts. You will be able to create hundreds of different routines using a jump rope, stability ball, resistance band, dumbbells, medicine ball and barbells. With the exception of the barbells, all of these items are portable and can be used anywhere—even outside, which helps keeps your routines interesting—and not confined to a gym or fitness center.

WORKOUT 1

Welcome to the Level III workouts! They allow you to move ahead, enjoying even higher levels of energy and endurance, greater loss of body fat, more flexibility, and increased muscular tone and strength. These workouts are tailored for individuals who like to work out at the gym or who have a medicine ball, dumbbells, barbells and a sturdy bench in their home gym.

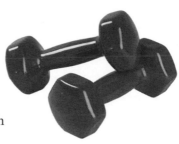

4 minutes | High-Energy Aerobic Training

Mountain Climber/ Jogging in Place

EQUIPMENT: **None (Optional: exercise mat)**
MUSCLES WORKED: **Heart, shoulders, core and legs**

Mountain climbing is a challenging activity that requires superior cardiovascular health, endurance, strength, agility and coordination—not to mention mental focus. If climbing up a steep, cold, treacherous mountain at terrifying heights is not something you plan to do in the near future, I'd like to show you a safe, convenient alternative. This challenging aerobic activity tones and strengthens every muscle in your body in a one-of-a-kind floor exercise. (If you haven't warmed up, start with a moderate jog.) Are you ready to meet me at the top? I've always wanted to say that!

▶ GET STARTED

Assume a push-up position: arms extended, hands shoulder-width apart, legs straight and heels up. Tilt your head slightly up and look forward toward the floor. (**Position 1**)

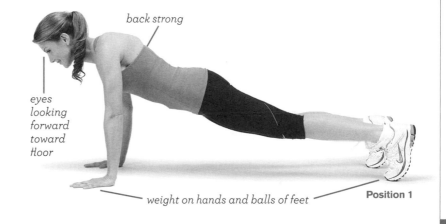

back strong

eyes looking forward toward floor

weight on hands and balls of feet

Position 1

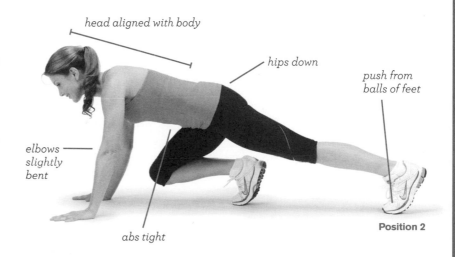

head aligned with body

hips down

push from balls of feet

elbows slightly bent

abs tight

Position 2

LEVEL III

187

Next, bring your right knee underneath your chest, distributing your weight between your hands, the ball of your right foot beneath you and the ball of your left foot behind you. (**Position 2**)

▶ GET MOVING

1. Keeping your elbows slightly bent, kick your right leg straight back behind you while simultaneously drawing your left knee and foot up toward your chest. Continue alternating legs at a moderate pace to warm up your muscles. To get the most out of this exercise, push off from the balls of your feet, moving as quickly as you can, and drive your knees up toward your chest. Keep your abdominal muscles tight, your hips low and your head in alignment with your body. Imagine you're climbing a mountain that just happens to be underneath you. Perform this exercise for 30 seconds.

2. Next, stand up and begin the Jogging in Place movements at a moderate pace. (**Position 3**) Remember to bring your hands from your hips up to your shoulders and then back. After jogging for 30 seconds, assume the Mountain Climber position and get ready to do it again—only faster this time. The first couple of minutes should be used to warm up your body, so remember to ease into your workout, increasing your pace as you progress through the 4 minutes.

3. Continue to alternate moderate Jogging in Place with intense "mountain climbing" every 30 seconds, for a total of 4 minutes. See if your Jogging in Place can progressively become somewhat faster and your "mountain climbing" periods can get quite a bit faster.

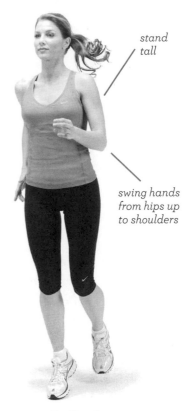

stand tall

swing hands from hips up to shoulders

Position 3

Too hard? Tone it down
- Perform both exercises more slowly.
- Perform the Mountain Climber with your hands placed on a bench that is 6 to 12 inches high.
- March in place instead of jogging.
- Keep your hands on your hips while you jog.

Too easy? Kick it up
- Perform both exercises more rapidly.
- Instead of jogging, alternate moderate and rapid "mountain climbing" every 30 seconds.
- Bring your knees farther up, closer to your chest.
- Perform this exercise for a longer period of time.

TAKE 10 TIPS

Think of being "light on your feet" as you alternate feet during the Mountain Climber. Also, throughout the exercise, keep your back straight and abs tight and strong. Way to go! You made it to the top!

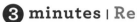

3 minutes | Resistance Exercise

Dumbbell Squat, Curl and Press

EQUIPMENT: 2 dumbbells

MUSCLES WORKED: Legs, butt, arms, shoulders and core

This is one of my favorite "fitness fusion" exercises, as it combines three separate movements: a squat, an arm curl and a shoulder press in rapid succession, using dumbbells.* You'll feel this exercise everywhere—it helps tone and shape your entire body!

❯ GET STARTED

Holding a dumbbell in each hand by the sides of your legs, stand with your knees slightly bent and your feet shoulder-width apart.

❯ GET MOVING

1. Sit back into a squat position by slowly lowering your weight as if you were going to sit in a chair. Keeping your chest up, your shoulders relaxed and your abdominal muscles tight, go down as low as you comfortably can. Remember to look straight ahead and to keep your toes in front of your knees. You should be able to draw an imaginary vertical line from your knee to the middle of your foot. (**Position 1**)

2. Next, tighten the muscles of your buttocks and straighten to a standing position, pushing from both heels. Then, keeping your knees slightly bent, rotate your hands so the dumbbells are in front of your thighs. Your elbows should be close to your sides and your palms facing away from your body. Slightly curl your wrists toward your forearms to prevent undue strain. Next, bending both arms and tightening your biceps, raise the dumbbells up toward your shoulders. Keep your wrists firm and strong. Hold the dumbbells near the front of your shoulders for 2 seconds. This is the arm curl part of the exercise. (**Position 2**)

When selecting a dumbbell or barbell, pick a weight you can safely use for 10 to 12 repetitions. Too heavy? Decrease the weight by 2 to 5 pounds, or as much as necessary to allow you to perform an exercise with proper form for at least 10 to 12 repetitions. Too light? If you can perform any dumbbell or barbell exercise with proper form for 12 reps without challenging your muscles, increase the weight by 2 to 5 pounds (or more); however, never sacrifice proper lifting technique for the sake of increasing the intensity of an exercise.

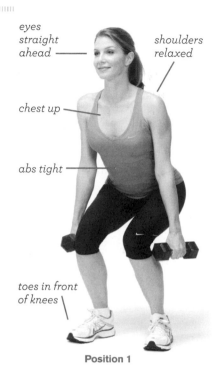

eyes straight ahead

shoulders relaxed

chest up

abs tight

toes in front of knees

Position 1

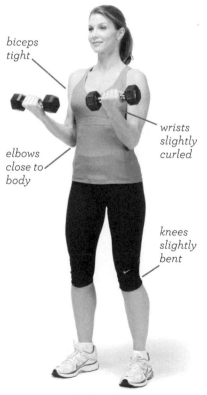

biceps tight

wrists slightly curled

elbows close to body

knees slightly bent

Position 2

LEVEL III

189

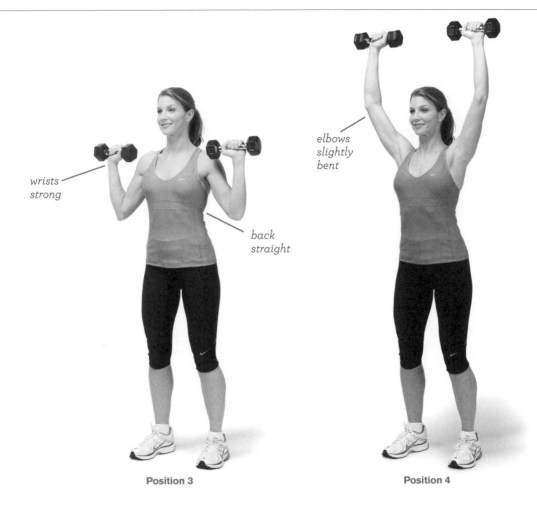

wrists strong

back straight

elbows slightly bent

Position 3

Position 4

3. Rotate the dumbbells again, so your palms are facing away from you and the backs of your knuckles are level with your shoulders. (**Position 3**) Keeping your wrists strong, extend your arms up in the air, pressing the dumbbells up and together above your head; hold this position for 2 seconds. Imagine someone just said, "Stick 'em up!" Stand straight, and keep your elbows slightly bent. This is the shoulder press part of the exercise. (**Position 4**) Slowly lower the dumbbells back to shoulder level, then back down to your sides.

4. Repeat this exercise as many times as you can for up to 1 minute.

TAKE 10 TIPS

Make sure your back is tall and strong throughout the exercise. Also, keep your head in alignment with your body. Remember to look straight ahead and to breathe comfortably throughout the exercise.

Too hard? Tone it down
- Start with a quarter-squat.
- Decrease the weight of the dumbbells.
- Perform this exercise for less than 1 minute.

Too easy? Kick it up
- Go lower into your squat.
- Hold the squat position for a longer period of time.
- Raise one dumbbell at a time when performing the shoulder press.
- Do a one-legged shoulder press. After you've pushed up out of the squat

position and done your curl, stand on one foot while raising the dumbbells over your head. Keep performing the movement, alternating legs.
- Increase the weight of the dumbbells.
- Perform this exercise for more than 1 minute.

LEVEL III

190

Dumbbell Swing

EQUIPMENT: **1 dumbbell**

MUSCLES WORKED: **Legs, butt, shoulder, arms and core**

We are bringing swing back into fashion—not in a dance, but in an exercise. The Dumbbell Swing, which involves "swinging" a dumbbell from the ground up toward your head, is a total body exercise. Be sure you're doing it safely and correctly.

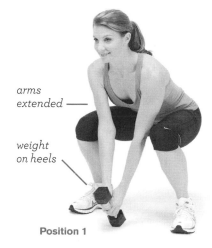

arms extended

weight on heels

Position 1

▶ GET STARTED

Place a dumbbell on its end on the floor in front of you. Stand with your feet a little wider than shoulder-width apart, toes pointed slightly out to the side. Squat down and firmly grab the dumbbell with both hands. You should be able to draw an imaginary vertical line from your knees to the middle of your feet. This is your starting position. (**Position 1**)

▶ GET MOVING

1. With your chest up, arms extended and elbows slightly bent, grasp the dumbbell with both hands. Keeping your abdominal muscles tight, press both feet to the floor, thrust your hips forward and stand up while swinging the dumbbell to shoulder level. Your back should be straight, your shoulders relaxed and your chin parallel to the floor. (**Position 2**)

2. Keeping your arms extended, lower the dumbbell slowly down between your legs, bending your knees and resuming your starting squat position.

3. Perform as many repetitions as you can in 1 minute.

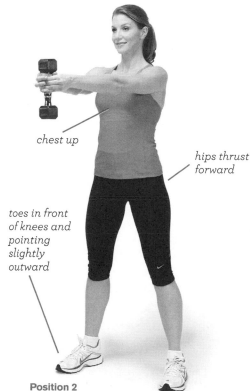

chest up

hips thrust forward

toes in front of knees and pointing slightly outward

Position 2

Too hard? Tone it down
- Decrease the weight of the dumbbell.
- Start with a quarter-squat.
- Don't swing the dumbbell as high.
- Take a rest between repetitions.

Too easy? Kick it up
- Increase the weight of the dumbbell.
- Go lower in your squat.
- Raise the dumbbell above your head.
- Hold the dumbbell with one hand. Perform the exercise with one arm at a time, alternating sides. Keep your other hand on your hip or by your side.
- Perform the exercise for longer than 1 minute.

TAKE 10 TIPS

When performing the Dumbbell Swing, think of your arms as a pendulum. Throughout the exercise, your head should be aligned with your body. Look straight ahead, and be sure your abs are tight and your back is straight.

LEVEL III

Dumbbell Side Shoulder Raise with Step Up

EQUIPMENT: 2 dumbbells and bench 8 to 18 inches high
MUSCLES WORKED: Legs, butt, core and shoulders

This exercise incorporates a shoulder motion and a step-up motion, using a bench and dumbbells. This is a great exercise to perform in a gym or outside in a park near a bench, picnic table or some steps.

▶ GET STARTED

Facing the bench, with your feet hip-width apart and your knees slightly bent, hold a dumbbell in each hand at the sides of your body. Your palms should be facing your sides. Next, place your right foot on top of the bench. (**Position 1**)

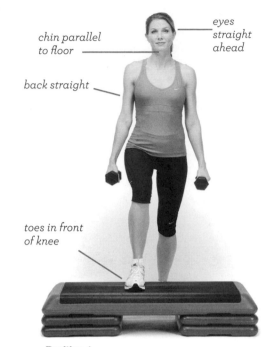

eyes straight ahead
chin parallel to floor
back straight
toes in front of knee

Position 1

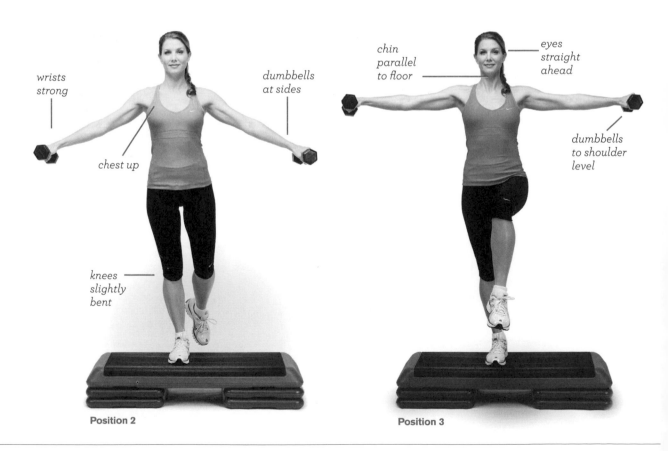

wrists strong
dumbbells at sides
chest up
knees slightly bent

Position 2

chin parallel to floor
eyes straight ahead
dumbbells to shoulder level

Position 3

LEVEL III

❯ GET MOVING

1. With dumbbells by your sides, push up and forward into a standing position on top of the bench, pressing from the heel of your right foot and the ball of your left foot. As you stand, place your body weight on your right foot allowing your left foot to be near or touching the top of the bench. (**Position 2**)

2. Next, with your back straight and your chin parallel to the floor, raise your left leg in front of you while lifting the dumbbells out away from your body and up to shoulder level (or as high as you can manage). Hold for 2 seconds. (**Position 3**) (Note: If you feel too unbalanced in this position, balance your weight by bringing your left foot more firmly on top of the bench. The wider your stance the more balanced you'll feel.)

3. Slowly lower the dumbbells back down to your sides while bringing your left foot back down to the ground. Keep your right foot firmly planted on top of the bench.

Repeat this sequence as many times as you can with the right foot on the bench for 30 seconds, then with the left leg as many times as you can for an additional 30 seconds.

Too hard? Tone it down

- Decrease the weight of the dumbbell.
- Perform the side shoulder raise while standing in front of the bench, before stepping up.
- Alternate legs when performing the step-up.
- Select a lower bench or step.
- Don't raise the dumbbells as high when performing the Side Shoulder Raise.
- Perform this exercise for a shorter period of time.

Too easy? Kick it up

- Increase the weight of the dumbbell.
- Select a higher bench or step.
- Raise the dumbbells in front of your body. Follow the instructions above, but start with the dumbbells near your thighs, with your palms facing your body. Do the shoulder raise to the front, lifting the dumbbells to shoulder level.
- While holding the dumbbells at shoulder level, slowly raise the left knee toward your waist, tightening your abs and keeping your wrists strong. Hold this position at the highest point for 2 seconds.
- Perform this exercise for longer than 1 minute.

TAKE 10 TIPS

Move at a slow and controlled pace throughout this exercise. Keep looking straight ahead of you, since looking down at your feet can affect your balance. And remember to breathe comfortably.

LEVEL III

2 minutes | Core-Strengthening Exercises

Dumbbell Twist

EQUIPMENT: 1 dumbbell
MUSCLES WORKED: Core (waist, lower back and abs)

This unique core movement has also been referred to as the Russian Twist in the athletic world. I believe the name comes from its popularity in Russia for training elite athletes competing in the Olympic Games. The good news: You don't have to be an elite athlete to perform this exercise, nor do you have to be Russian!

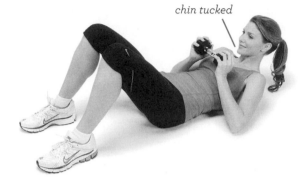

chin tucked

Position 1

▶ GET STARTED

Begin this exercise by lying on your back, shoulders relaxed, knees bent and feet flat on the floor hip-width apart. Hold a dumbbell horizontally in both hands close to the middle of your chest. Tuck your chin toward your chest as if you're holding an orange under your chin. (**Position 1**)

▶ GET MOVING

1. Tightening your abdominal muscles and bending from the waist, draw your shoulders and upper back off the floor. Ideally your torso will be at a 45° angle to the floor. Extend both arms and hold the dumbbell in front of your chest. (**Position 2**)

2. Now, while your shoulders and upper back are off the floor, slowly rotate your upper torso as far as you comfortably can to the left, still holding the dumbbell in both hands and keeping your arms equally extended. Begin this motion from the waist, and move your head with your torso. (**Position 3**) Hold the twist for 2 seconds, then slowly rotate your shoulders and arms to the other side. Hold for another 2 seconds.

3. Alternate sides as many times as you can for up to 1 minute.

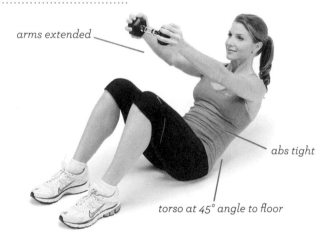

arms extended

abs tight

torso at 45° angle to floor

Position 2

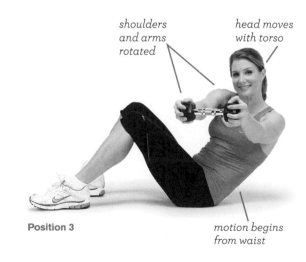

shoulders and arms rotated

head moves with torso

motion begins from waist

Position 3

LEVEL III

Too hard? Tone it down

- Decrease the weight of the dumbbell— or practice without using a dumbbell.
- Perform this motion without raising your shoulders and upper back off the floor.
- Bend your arms when rotating to the sides. The closer the dumbbell is to your chest, the easier this movement will be.
- Rest between rotations.
- Hold the twist for less than 2 seconds.
- Perform the exercise for less than 1 minute.

Too easy? Kick it up

- Increase the weight of the dumbbell.
- Move more slowly.
- Hold the twist for more than 2 seconds.
- Perform this exercise for longer than 1 minute.

Leg Tucked Dumbbell Crunch

EQUIPMENT: **1 dumbbell**
MUSCLES WORKED: **Core (abs)**

You're about to take firming and strengthening your abs to the next level. By adding a dumbbell for resistance and holding your legs off the ground, you create a great variation on a regular crunch. You can alter the difficulty of this movement just by changing the way you hold the dumbbell.

> **GET STARTED**

Begin this exercise by lying on your back with your feet off the floor and your calves tucked close to the backs of your thighs. Hold a dumbbell horizontally across your chest, with your hands on each side of the dumbbell, close to your chin. Next, tuck your chin toward your chest, raising your head off the floor. Imagine you're holding an orange under your chin. (**Position 1**)

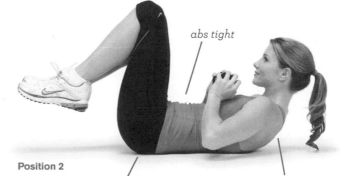

calves tucked

dumbbell close to chin

chin tucked

head raised

Position 1

abs tight

Position 2

lower back pressed to floor

upper back off the floor

❯ GET MOVING

1. Tighten your abdominal muscles and roll your shoulders and upper back off the floor. As you exhale, raise up toward your knees. Come up as far as you can while keeping the small of your lower back pressed to the floor. (**Position 2**) Hold the crunch for 2 seconds, then return slowly toward the floor. Touch your upper back to the floor and quickly rise up again.

2. Perform this movement as many times as you can for up to 1 minute.

Too hard? Tone it down
- Decrease the weight of the dumbbell.
- Practice this movement without a dumbbell.
- Don't raise your shoulders as high off the floor.
- Lie on the floor between repetitions.
- Hold the crunch for a shorter period of time.
- Perform this exercise for less than 1 minute.

Too easy? Kick it up
- Increase the weight of the dumbbell.
- Hold the dumbbell over your chest with your arms extended straight out, elbows slightly bent.
- Hold the dumbbell over your head, arms extended, and elbows slightly bent.
- Extend your legs straight up in the air, knees slightly bent and heels facing the sky.
- Hold the crunch for longer than 2 seconds.
- Perform this exercise for longer than 1 minute.

> **TAKE 10 TIPS**
>
> To get the most out of this abdominal exercise, tighten your abs as you lift the dumbbell toward your knees and raise your shoulders off the floor.

① minute | Stretching and Deep Breathing

Side Lunge Stretch

EQUIPMENT: None

MUSCLES WORKED: Butt and inner thighs

Here's a stretch you can perform anytime, anywhere—at home brushing your teeth or in the shower, or at work on the phone. You don't need any special equipment, and best of all, you can perform it from a standing position.

❯ GET STARTED

With your chest up and shoulders relaxed, stand tall with your feet wider than shoulder-width apart, toes pointing forward. The wider your stance, the greater your stretch will be. Place your hands on your hips. (**Position 1**)

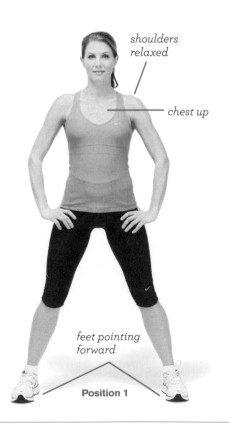

shoulders relaxed

chest up

feet pointing forward

Position 1

❯ GET MOVING

1. Pointing your right foot slightly out to the side, bend your right leg until your knee is directly over the ball of your right foot. Be sure your knee does not extend over your toes. Keep your chest up and your head in an upright position as you look straight ahead. On the other side, keep your left leg as straight as you can. Once you arrive at a distance where you experience a stretch in the inner thigh of the straightened leg, hold the stretch and breathe deeply. (**Position 2**)

2. Hold this stretch for 15 seconds, then switch legs, point the other foot to the side and stretch to the other side for another 15 seconds.

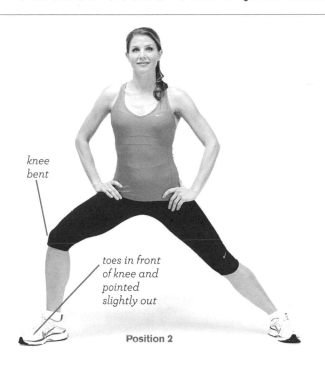

knee bent

toes in front of knee and pointed slightly out

Position 2

Too hard? Tone it down
- Decrease the distance of your stretch.
- Hold this stretch for a shorter period of time.

Too easy? Kick it up
- Increase the distance of your stretch.
- Push your hip forward to increase the stretch.
- Hold the stretch for a longer period of time.

TAKE 10 TIPS

To get the most out of this stretch, turn the toes of the bent leg slightly out to the side. This little motion opens up your hips to increase the range of the stretch.

Seated Hip Stretch

EQUIPMENT: Chair or bench
MUSCLES WORKED: Lower back and hips

People who can sit cross-legged with ease have great flexibility of the knee joints and hip area. This is a fantastic stretch to increase the flexibility of your lower back, hips and knee joints. You can perform it anywhere you'd like—all you need is a chair or bench to sit on.

❯ GET STARTED

Sit on a chair or bench with your chest up and both feet on the floor, hip-width apart. While sitting up straight, place your right foot and ankle on top of your left knee/thigh.

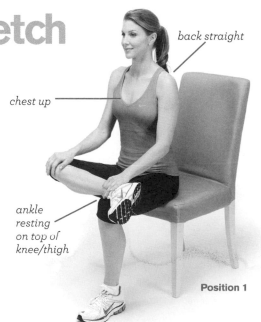

back straight

chest up

ankle resting on top of knee/thigh

Position 1

Place your right hand on top of your right knee, and grasp your right ankle (on top of your left knee) with your left hand. (**Position 1**)

▶ GET MOVING

1. While keeping your back straight and shoulders relaxed, bend forward from the waist, lowering your chest and shoulders. Keep your head in alignment with your torso. At the same time, apply gentle pressure with your right hand on top of your right knee. (**Position 2**) You should feel the stretch in your hip and lower back.

2. Breathing deeply, hold this stretch for 15 seconds. Then relax and come back up to a sitting position. Switch legs and perform the stretch on the other side for another 15 seconds.

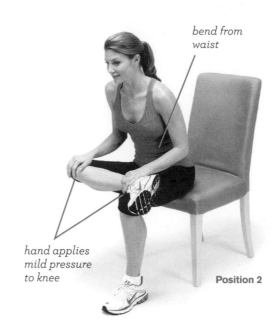

bend from waist

hand applies mild pressure to knee

Position 2

Too hard? Tone it down
- Decrease the depth of your stretch.
- Hold the stretch for a shorter period of time.

Too easy? Kick it up
- Increase the depth of your stretch.
- Hold the stretch for a longer period of time.
- Place your foot higher up on your thigh.

TAKE 10 TIPS

To get the most out of this exercise, remember to bend forward from the waist and gently apply slight pressure on the crossed leg to enhance the stretch.

Well done!
You have just completed your first 4•3•2•1 workout at Level III! Now you can stop and give yourself a high-five, or go back and repeat parts of this workout or the entire circuit.

LEVEL III

WORKOUT 2

This workout introduces a new item to your fitness regimen that is actually one of the oldest and most versatile pieces of fitness equipment ever used: the medicine ball. In this workout I've put together some challenging moves that will get you fit fast, making you stronger, leaner and healthier—quicker!

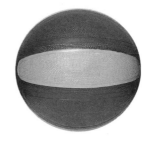

4 minutes | High-Energy Aerobic Training

Jumping Lunge

EQUIPMENT: **None (Optional: exercise mat)**
MUSCLES WORKED: **Heart, shoulders, hips, butt and legs**

What do you think is the number one aerobic activity for burning calories and improving overall fitness? There are many exercises to choose from, but none can compare to cross-country skiing, which involves every major muscle group. For this exercise, you will imitate this sports activity—but without the equipment and the subzero temperatures! Your starting position is a split lunge, but then you will alternate legs as quickly as you can, jumping from one leg to the other while moving your arms back and forth as if you were pushing with ski poles. All you need is a little space and you're on your way.

❯ GET STARTED

Begin this motion by standing in a split-lunge position, about a quarter of the way down, knees slightly bent and your weight divided between the heel of your right foot in front and the ball of your left foot in back. Swing your left hand up, with your right hand and arm down by your right thigh. (**Position 1**)

❯ GET MOVING

1. Tighten your abdominal muscles and jump straight up in the air, pushing from the balls of both feet, alternating your legs like scissors in midair. Simultaneously, switch arms. Thrust your right hand up and lower your left arm to your thigh. (**Position 2**)

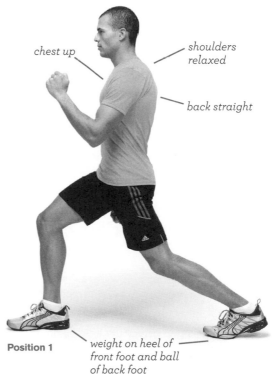

chest up

shoulders relaxed

back straight

Position 1

weight on heel of front foot and ball of back foot

LEVEL III

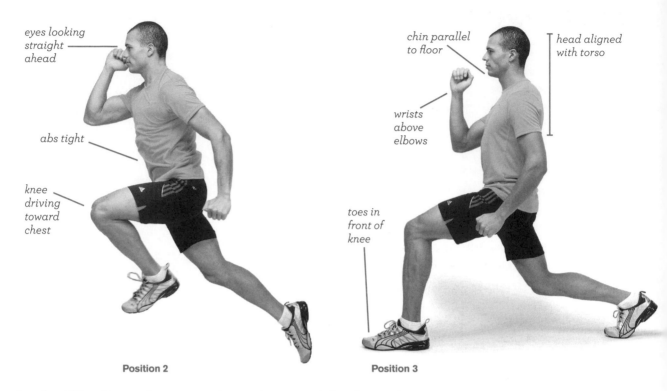

eyes looking straight ahead

abs tight

knee driving toward chest

chin parallel to floor

head aligned with torso

wrists above elbows

toes in front of knee

Position 2

Position 3

You should land in another quarter-lunge. (**Position 3**) Continue to jump, alternating arms and legs, at a moderate pace for 30 seconds. Remember to keep your chest up and your shoulders relaxed. The first couple of minutes should be used to warm up your body, so remember to ease into your workout, increasing your pace as you progress through the 4 minutes.

2. Now perform the same motion, but go faster and do a full lunge as you land. Your front thigh should be parallel to the floor with your toes in front of your knee. Keep your back straight, your head aligned with your body and your chin parallel to the floor. Keep moving your arms and legs as fast as you comfortably can for 30 seconds.

3. Alternate slow and fast Jumping Lunges every 30 seconds for a total of 4 minutes. See if your "slow" periods can progressively become a little faster and your "fast" periods can get quite a bit faster.

TAKE 10 TIPS

To get the most out of this exercise, remember to push off from the balls of your feet, moving as quickly as you can. Think of being light on your feet as you alternate arms and legs. Also, be sure your toes are in front of your knee in the lunge position.

Too hard? Tone it down
- Move more slowly throughout this exercise.
- Place your hands on your hips throughout the exercise.
- Jump lower.
- Keep doing quarter-lunges instead of trying to go deeper.

- During the "slow" 30 seconds, march in place instead of doing Jumping Lunges.
- Perform this exercise for a shorter period of time.

Too easy? Kick it up
- Move more quickly throughout the exercise.
- Go deeper in your lunges.
- Jump higher.
- Exaggerate your arm motions, with big arm swings.
- Perform this movement for a longer period of time.

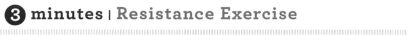

3 minutes | Resistance Exercise

Medicine Ball Overhead Squat

EQUIPMENT: Medicine ball

MUSCLES WORKED: Legs, butt, arms, shoulders, core, upper and lower back

In this movement, which tones and strengthens the entire body, you'll be performing a squat while holding a medicine ball* over your head the entire time. This provides an added challenge—your abs, upper and lower back, shoulders, arms, butt and legs work overtime trying to hold up the medicine ball and keep your body in balance. After performing this Medicine Ball Overhead Squat, you'll probably agree that 1 minute is enough!

❯ GET STARTED

Hold the medicine ball with both hands in front of you below your waist with your arms extended, elbows slightly bent. Stand tall with your chest up, shoulders back and feet shoulder-width apart. Point your toes slightly out to the sides for balance. Next, with your back straight, raise the medicine ball over your head (the ball actually should be slightly behind your head), with both arms extended and elbows slightly bent. This is your starting position. (**Position 1**)

❯ GET MOVING

1. Tighten your abdominal muscles and sit back into a squat position by slowly lowering your weight down as if you were going to sit in a chair. Due to the weight of the medicine ball, it is natural to lean forward slightly from the waist as you maintain your balance, so try to keep the medicine ball as far back as you can as you lower down into the squat position, pushing back with your arms and shoulders.

When selecting a medicine ball, pick a weight you can safely use for 10 to 12 repetitions. Too heavy? Decrease the weight by 2 to 5 pounds, or as much as necessary to allow you to perform an exercise with proper form for at least 10 to 12 repetitions. Too light? If you can perform any medicine ball exercise with proper form for 12 reps without challenging your muscles, increase the weight by 2 to 5 pounds (or more); however, never sacrifice proper technique for the sake of increasing the intensity of an exercise.

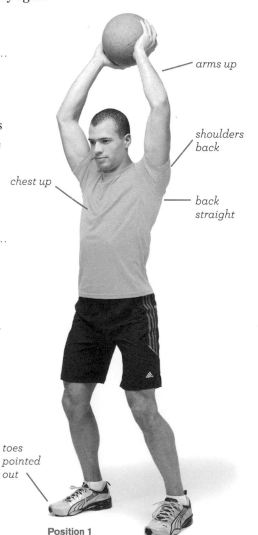

arms up

shoulders back

chest up

back straight

toes pointed out

Position 1

Your toes should be in front of your knees so that you could draw imaginary vertical lines from your knees to the middle of your feet. Go down as low as you comfortably can. Keep your chest up, look straight ahead and hold the medicine ball above your head throughout this motion, keeping your wrists firm and strong. (**Position 2**)

2. Next, tighten the muscles of your buttocks and push up to a standing position, pressing from the heels of both feet. Keep the medicine ball over your head, with both arms extended and elbows slightly bent.

3. Keeping your torso straight, perform this exercise as many times as you can for up to 1 minute.

Too hard? Tone it down

- Choose a lighter medicine ball.
- Start with a quarter-squat.
- Perform the exercise without a medicine ball, but hold your hands over your head for practice.
- Lower the medicine ball down to your waist as you stand up.
- Rest between repetitions.
- Perform this exercise for less than 1 minute.

Too easy? Kick it up

- Choose a heavier medicine ball.
- Go lower into your squat.
- Hold the squat position for a longer period of time.
- Perform this movement for more than 1 minute.

TAKE 10 TIPS

Keeping your chest up will help you keep the ball overhead. Also, choosing a medicine ball that is too heavy won't make you stronger—it will just ruin your form. Remember to keep your head in alignment with your body as you look straight ahead and to breathe comfortably throughout the exercise.

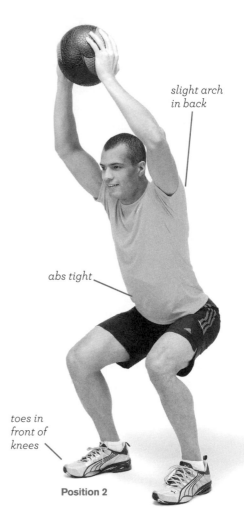

slight arch in back

abs tight

toes in front of knees

Position 2

Medicine Ball Knee Push-Up

EQUIPMENT: Medicine ball
MUSCLES WORKED: Chest, shoulders, arms and core

Now it's time to incorporate a medicine ball into one of the most challenging upper body exercises: the push-up. Like the other exercises in this workout, this motion challenges your entire body and can be done anywhere. Balancing one hand and arm on the medicine ball forces your chest, shoulder, arms and core to work harder. For this exercise, using a larger medicine ball makes the Knee Push-Up more challenging, since a larger medicine ball increases the range of motion in the shoulder and chest muscles; conversely, a smaller medicine ball decreases the range of motion. I usually recommend beginning this exercise with an 8- to 10-pound smooth medicine ball with no handles. Be sure to select the ball best suited for your level of fitness.

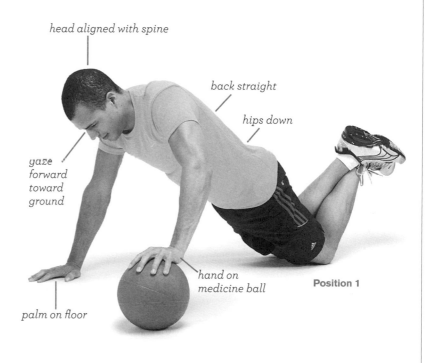

head aligned with spine

back straight

hips down

gaze forward toward ground

palm on floor

hand on medicine ball

Position 1

▶ GET STARTED

Position yourself on the floor with your left hand on the medicine ball slightly out to the side. Keep your back straight, looking forward toward the floor with your head in alignment with your spine. Next, raise your heels toward your butt at a 45° angle and cross your ankles. Keep your knees firmly on the floor and your hips down. This is your starting position. (**Position 1**)

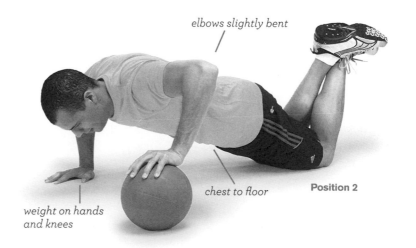

elbows slightly bent

chest to floor

weight on hands and knees

Position 2

LEVEL III

203

❯ GET MOVING

1. Next, lower your chest slowly toward the floor by bending both elbows, going as low as you comfortably can with the goal of trying to touch your chin to the ground. Remember to tighten your abdominal muscles and to keep your back straight. Ideally, you will perform this motion without your upper thighs touching the ground, which places more weight on your knees and hands. (**Position 2**)

2. Perform this exercise as many times as you can with your left arm on the medicine ball for 30 seconds, then switch arms for an additional 30 seconds.

Too hard? Tone it down

- Instead of touching your chin to the ground, go down only a quarter of the way. Gradually increase the depth of your push-ups as you become stronger.
- Allow your thighs to touch the ground as you lower down.
- Go at your own pace. As your muscles become better conditioned, you will increase the pace and your total number of repetitions.
- Use a smaller medicine ball.

Too easy? Kick it up

- Lower your upper body as far as you can. The lower you go, the more challenging the exercise will be for your arms, chest and shoulders.
- Place your hands closer together.
- Uncross your ankles, extend the leg opposite the medicine ball and raise it off the floor while you perform your push-ups. Switch sides after 30 seconds.
- Perform a one-handed Medicine Ball Knee Push-Up (these are tough!). Place one hand on the medicine ball and the other behind your back.

- Use a classic or military push-up position. Uncross your ankles, extend both legs and balance your weight on the medicine ball, the palm of the other hand and the balls of your feet, with your feet positioned hip-width apart.
- After each push-up, alternate hands on the medicine ball. When you're in the extended push-up position, roll the medicine ball under your torso to the opposite side, then place your other hand on top of the ball.
- Place both hands on top of the medicine ball under your chest and perform knee push-ups.
- Place both hands on top of the medicine ball under your chest and perform military push-ups with your legs extended and your weight on your hands and the balls of your feet.
- Use a larger medicine ball.
- Perform the push-ups explosively.

TAKE 10 TIPS

To get the most out of this exercise, keep your abs tight and your back straight. Remember to exhale as you push away from the floor and breathe comfortably throughout the exercise. Press the medicine ball into the floor—you don't want it to roll when you're pushing up.

Medicine Ball Walking Lunge with a Twist

EQUIPMENT: Medicine ball

MUSCLES WORKED: Legs, butt, shoulders and core (abs and waist)

This exercise takes the traditional "walking lunge" motion to an entirely new level. Here you get to experience a new way of incorporating motions for the upper body, core and lower body all in one exercise. This will test your strength, flexibility, balance and stamina all at the same time. Select a medicine ball that allows you to perform the exercise with proper form and technique. I generally recommend beginning this exercise with a lighter (3- to 5-pound) medicine ball.

▶ GET STARTED

Stand with your feet hip-width apart, knees slightly bent, holding the medicine ball at your chest with both hands. Look straight ahead. This is your starting position. (**Position 1**)

▶ GET MOVING

1. Start with a split-lunge position. Step forward 2 to 3 feet with your right foot, balancing your weight between the heel of your right foot in front and the ball of your left foot in back. Next, lower your right thigh until it's parallel to the floor (or as low as you can manage). Make sure you don't extend your knee over your toes when in the lunge position; if you find yourself in this position, take a longer lunge step and adjust your stance. You should be able to draw an imaginary vertical line between your front knee and the middle of your front foot. Lower your left knee down to the floor without actually touching it. As you lower down in the lunge motion, extend both arms in front of you, elbows slightly bent, holding the medicine ball at chest level away from your body. (**Position 2**)

2. Now rotate the medicine ball to the right as far as you comfortably can. Begin this rotation from the waist, and move your head, shoulders, arms and torso as one unit. Keep your chin parallel to the floor, your shoulders relaxed and your chest up. (**Position 3**)

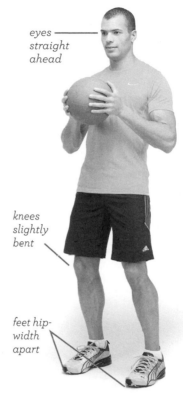

eyes straight ahead

knees slightly bent

feet hip-width apart

Position 1

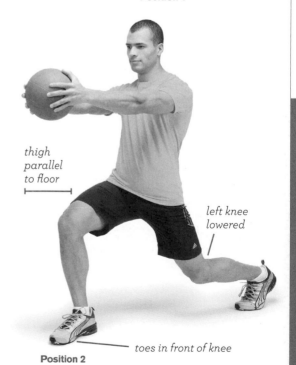

thigh parallel to floor

left knee lowered

toes in front of knee

Position 2

LEVEL III

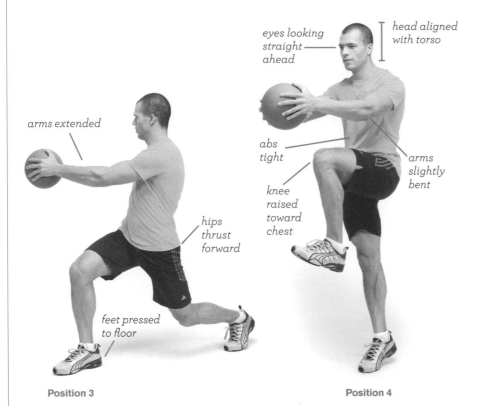

arms extended

hips thrust forward

feet pressed to floor

Position 3

eyes looking straight ahead

head aligned with torso

abs tight

knee raised toward chest

arms slightly bent

Position 4

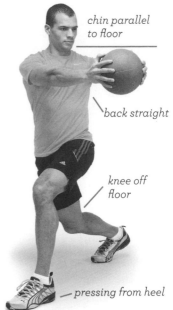

chin parallel to floor

back straight

knee off floor

pressing from heel

Position 5

3. Next, pressing from the heel of your right foot in front and the ball of your left foot in back, tighten your abdominal muscles and push up and forward, walking into your next lunge position with your left thigh parallel to the floor. (**Position 4**) Rotate the medicine ball to the other side. (**Position 5**)

4. Continue your walking lunges, rotating the medicine ball back and forth, as many times as you can for up to 1 minute.

Too hard? Tone it down

- When you rotate your torso, hold the medicine ball closer to your chest, with your arms bent. The closer the ball is to your body, the easier the exercise.
- Perform this movement without a medicine ball, but hold something small like a tennis ball for practice.
- Use quarter-lunges, bending your front and back legs slightly.
- Rest between repetitions.

Too easy? Kick it up

- Use a heavier medicine ball.
- Go lower in your lunge.
- As you transition between lunges, raise your back leg up to your chest and hold. Then step down into your lunge motion.

TAKE 10 TIPS

Throughout this exercise, keep your back straight and your shoulders relaxed, move at a slow and controlled pace, and breathe comfortably.

② minutes | Core-Strengthening Exercises

Medicine Ball Slam

EQUIPMENT: Medicine ball
MUSCLES WORKED: Shoulders, abs, back and legs

If you're having a stressful day, there's no better exercise than this! It will help you get out any frustration while toning and strengthening your shoulders, abs, back and lower body at the same time. All you need is a medicine ball and a small area to slam away! Select a medicine ball that allows you to perform the exercise with proper form and technique. I generally recommend beginning this exercise with a lighter medicine ball (no more than 8 pounds).

▶ GET STARTED

Stand with your back straight, knees slightly bent and feet a little wider than shoulder-width apart. Hold a medicine ball with both hands over your head, arms extended, shoulders back and elbows slightly bent. (**Position 1**)

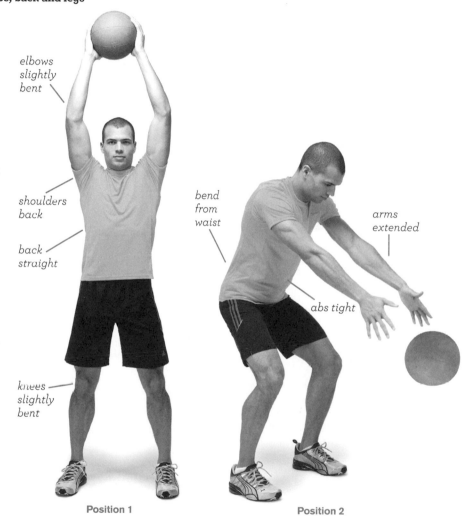

elbows slightly bent

shoulders back

back straight

knees slightly bent

bend from waist

arms extended

abs tight

Position 1

Position 2

▶ GET MOVING

1. With one powerful motion, tighten your abdominal muscles and slam the ball to the floor as hard as you can. Keep your arms extended, elbows slightly bent, and, bending from the waist, keep your head in alignment with your torso. (**Position 2**)

2. Squat down and grab the medicine ball (or catch it, if it bounces), stand back up and raise it over your head again, with arms extended, getting ready to repeat the motion.

3. Perform this movement as many times as you can for up to 1 minute.

LEVEL III

Too hard? Tone it down

- Use a lighter medicine ball.
- Raise the medicine ball to shoulder level instead of overhead.
- Rest between slams.
- Perform the exercise for less than 1 minute.

Too easy? Kick it up

- Use a heavier medicine ball.
- Slam the ball down from side to side instead of directly in front of you. Start with the ball high over your right shoulder and slam it down to the left side of your body.
- Move faster.
- Squat down lower when retrieving the medicine ball from the floor.
- Perform the exercise for longer than 1 minute.

> **TAKE 10 TIPS**
>
> Remember to tighten your abs as you slam the medicine ball down as hard as you can, moving quickly and powerfully.

Medicine Ball Reverse Chop

EQUIPMENT: **Medicine ball**

MUSCLES WORKED: **Legs, butt, shoulders, core and upper back**

You performed this exercise in Level II using a resistance band (this is the exercise in which you do a reverse chopping motion, from bottom to top), but now you'll be taking it to the next level by performing it with a medicine ball and adding a squat. In this exercise, you will pull the medicine ball up from the floor toward the opposite side of your body above your head. Select a medicine ball that allows you to perform the exercise correctly with proper form and technique. I generally recommend beginning this exercise with a lighter (3- to 5-pound) medicine ball.

> **GET STARTED** ....

Begin in a squat position, as if you were about to sit in a chair, with your back straight and your feet shoulder-width apart. Your toes should be in front of your knees, and you should be able to draw an imaginary line from your knee to the middle of your front foot. With both arms extended, elbows slightly bent, hold a medicine ball in both hands to the outside of your right knee. (**Position 1**)

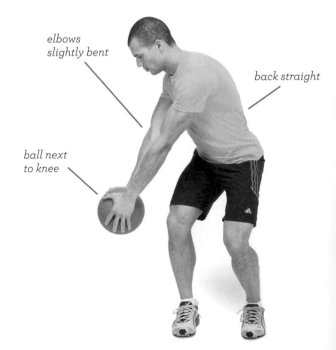

elbows slightly bent

back straight

ball next to knee

Position 1

LEVEL III

❯ GET MOVING

1. Come to a standing position, twisting the medicine ball across the front of your body until it's above your head and your arms are extended over your left shoulder. Move your head with your torso as you rotate your shoulders and hips, pivoting on the ball of your right foot. Initiate this movement from the waist, rather than swinging your arms and using the momentum of the medicine ball to complete the motion. (**Position 2**)

2. Slowly reverse the motion. Rotate your torso back to your original starting position, and bend your legs to a parallel squat.

3. Perform this movement as many times as you can for 30 seconds to one side, then repeat to the other side for an additional 30 seconds.

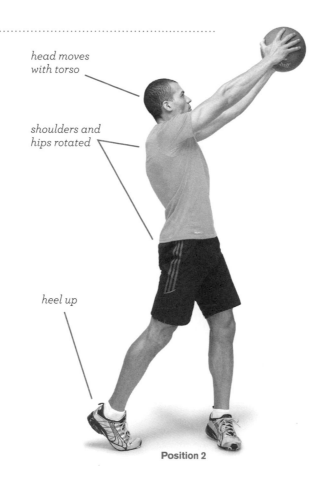

head moves with torso

shoulders and hips rotated

heel up

Position 2

Too hard? Tone it down

- Perform this movement without a medicine ball. Hold a tennis ball for practice.
- Begin with a quarter-squat.
- Don't reach as high when rotating your upper torso.
- Keep your arms bent throughout the entire exercise. Your rotation will be shorter.
- Perform the movement for less than 1 minute.

Too easy? Kick it up

- As you come back to the starting position, squat down as low as you can, reaching the medicine ball toward the ground.
- Choose a heavier medicine ball.
- Hold the medicine ball up as high as you can when rotating your upper torso.
- Vary your speed of movement. When twisting your body, rotate quickly, reaching up with the medicine ball above the side of your head. Rotate slowly back to your original squat position.
- Perform this exercise for longer than 1 minute.

TAKE 10 TIPS

To get the most out of this exercise, use your waist (oblique) muscles to twist your torso and to move slowly back down to the starting position.

LEVEL III

① minute | Stretching and Deep Breathing

Roll-Up

EQUIPMENT: Exercise mat or carpeted area
MUSCLES WORKED: Upper and lower back

Have you ever tumbled or done somersaults? Not recently, right? I want to show you a simple tumbling move so relaxing that it rolls all the kinks out of your back. No special equipment is needed—just your curiosity and willingness to be a kid again!

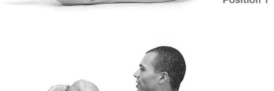

knees hugged

chin tucked

Position 1

▶ GET STARTED

Lying down on your back, draw both knees up toward your chest. Next, wrap both hands around your knees, drawing them as close to your chest as you can. Tuck your chin toward your chest as if you're holding an orange under your chin. (**Position 1**)

▶ GET MOVING

1. With your head tucked and knees close to your chest, slowly roll onto your lower back and butt, raising your upper back off the ground. (**Position 2**)

2. Next, with your head tucked and knees close to your chest, slowly roll back onto your shoulders and upper back, raising your buttocks off the floor. (**Position 3**)

3. Continue to rock gently back and forth without jerking, breathing comfortably, for 30 seconds.

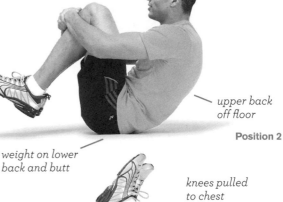

upper back off floor

Position 2

weight on lower back and butt

knees pulled to chest

buttocks off floor

weight on upper back and shoulders

Position 3

Too hard? Tone it down
- Hold your knees farther away from your chest.
- Perform this exercise for a shorter period of time.
- Don't try to roll as far.

Too easy? Kick it up
- Hold your knees and legs closer to your chest.
- Perform this exercise for a longer period of time.

TAKE 10 TIPS

To get the most out of this stretch, keep your chin tucked close to your chest and rock gently back and forth from the upper and lower positions. Remember to breathe deeply throughout the exercise and to move slowly and under control.

Lying Quad Stretch

EQUIPMENT: Exercise mat or carpeted area
MUSCLES WORKED: Fronts of legs (quads) and hips

Your last movement for this workout provides a soothing stretch to the quadriceps and hip muscles, increasing your flexibility and mobility. You can perform this stretch anywhere you'd like. All you need is a mat or a small piece of carpeted real estate where you can lie on your side.

▶ GET STARTED

Lie down on your left side with your body straight and your left arm under your head for support. (**Position 1**)

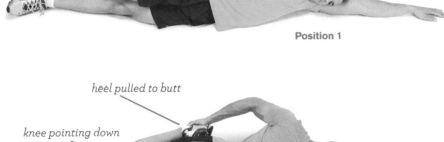

body straight

arm under head

Position 1

▶ GET MOVING

1. Bend your right leg and grab your ankle with your right hand. Slowly pull your heel toward your butt as you gently press the right side of your hip forward. Keep your left leg straight and your right knee down. (**Position 2**)

2. Hold this stretch for 15 seconds, then turn to the other side and perform the stretch for another 15 seconds.

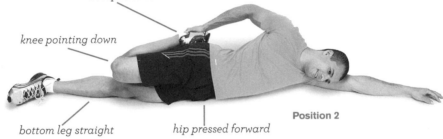

heel pulled to butt

knee pointing down

bottom leg straight

hip pressed forward

Position 2

Too hard? Tone it down
- If you're having difficulty holding the ankle of the bent leg, hold the back of your sock or shoe instead. As you perform this stretch more frequently, you'll be able to progress to holding your ankle.
- Don't stretch your leg so far.
- Hold the stretch for a shorter period of time.

Too easy? Kick it up
- Stretch your leg farther.
- Hold the stretch for a longer period of time.

TAKE 10 TIPS

To get the most out of this stretch, slowly rotate and press the hip of the stretched leg forward. Remember to breathe deeply as you perform this stretch.

LEVEL III

Well done!
You have just completed your second 4•3•2•1 workout at Level III!
Give yourself a reward, or go back and repeat sections of the workout or the entire circuit.

WORKOUT 3

Now you're ready to move ahead by incorporating barbells into your exercise routines. In Workout 3, you'll get the most out of your workouts with a "fast fitness" approach to barbell training. If you've used barbells before, note that I've put together some challenging moves that may not be familiar to you, so please read the instructions carefully.

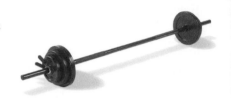

4 minutes | High-Energy Aerobic Training

Burpee (Squat Thrust) and Jogging in Place

EQUIPMENT: None (Optional: exercise mat)
MUSCLES WORKED: Heart, shoulders, arms, legs and core

Officially called the Squat Thrust, the Burpee has been a regular part of most phys ed programs for years. You probably want to say, "I did *not* like those when I was a kid!" but now that you're in Level III, you're more than ready to take the squat thrust out of the closet, dust it off and make it a regular part of your workouts. Often this exercise is called the Four-Count Burpee. If it helps you, count out **one** when you're standing with feet together, hands by your sides; **two** when you put your hands on the floor and thrust your feet back into a push-up position; **three** when you thrust your feet forward into the squat position again; and **four** when you stand back up. If you haven't warmed up, start with Jogging in Place.)

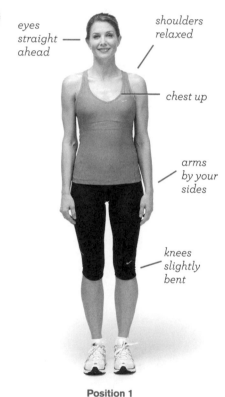

eyes straight ahead

shoulders relaxed

chest up

arms by your sides

knees slightly bent

Position 1

▶ GET STARTED

Stand with your arms by your sides, knees slightly bent and feet positioned hip-width apart. (Count **one!**) (**Position 1**)

▶ GET MOVING

1. Squat down and place your palms in front of your feet on the floor, looking down. (**Position 2**) Next, with your weight on your hands and your elbows slightly bent, thrust your feet back so you land in a classic push-up position. Your back should be straight, legs extended, and your weight divided between the palms of your hands and the balls of your feet. Keep your head in alignment with your body and look down, slightly in front of you. (Count **two!**) (**Position 3**)

knees bent

feet hip-width apart

palms in front of feet

Position 2

LEVEL III

2. Now thrust your feet forward, so you're back in the squat position. (Count **three**!) (**Position 2**) Then stand up straight again. (Count **four**!) (**Position 1**)

3. Perform this exercise at a leisurely pace, slowly and under control, to warm up your body for 30 seconds.

4. Next, stand up and begin to jog in place (see page 137) at a leisurely pace. Remember to bring your knees up and to swing your hands all the way from your hips up to your shoulders. After 30 seconds of light jogging, do another set of Burpees.

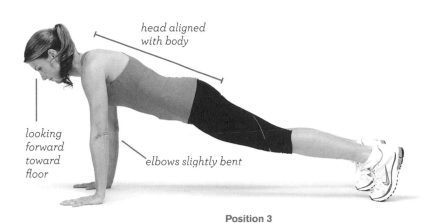

head aligned with body

looking forward toward floor

elbows slightly bent

Position 3

5. Keep alternating slow Jogging in Place with Burpees every 30 seconds for a total of 4 minutes. See if your "slow" jog periods can progressively become a little faster and your Burpees can get quite a bit faster. The first couple of minutes are used to warm up your body, so remember to increase your pace as you progress through the 4 minutes.

Too hard? Tone it down

- Move more slowly throughout the exercise.
- Squat only a quarter of the way down.
- March in place instead of jogging.
- Perform fewer repetitions.
- Perform this exercise for a shorter period of time.

Too easy? Kick it up

- Move your body more quickly throughout this exercise.
- Squat down lower.
- Instead of coming up out of your squat into a standing position, jump up in the air as high as you can and perform a jump squat. Then return to Position 1 and continue the exercise.
- Perform a push-up between the squats and thrusts.
- Perform more repetitions.
- Perform this exercise for a longer period of time.

TAKE 10 TIPS

When learning this exercise, don't do too many at first. Get used to doing the motions in the proper form, moving from standing to squatting to the push-up position, then back to squatting and standing again. When you feel you're performing the exercise correctly, increase your speed and intensity. After all, you're not a kid anymore!

LEVEL III

③ minutes | Resistance Exercise

Barbell Bench Press

EQUIPMENT: Barbell with weights and sturdy exercise bench
MUSCLES WORKED: Chest, shoulders and backs of arms (triceps)

For your first barbell exercise, you'll perform one of the most famous of all upper body resistance exercises: the Bench Press. Don't think this compound exercise is just for football players or musclemen. It's great for toning and strengthening your chest, shoulders and those tricky spots, the back of your arms. If you're bench-pressing a lot of weight, be sure to have someone "spot" you.

▶ GET STARTED

Lie on your back on a bench, with your head firmly supported (you should be looking at the ceiling) and both feet flat on the floor. With your wrists strong, grasp the bar with your hands shoulder-width apart on the bar, with both arms extended, elbows slightly bent. Wrap your thumbs around the bar. (**Position 1**)

▶ GET MOVING

1. Begin this exercise by inhaling and lowering the bar so that it's just touching the middle portion of your chest. (**Position 2**)

2. Next, still looking up at the ceiling, with your shoulders, upper back and hips pressed against the bench, press the bar up, driving both hands into the bar, exhaling and extending both arms back to the starting position.

3. Perform this exercise as many times as you can for up to 1 minute.

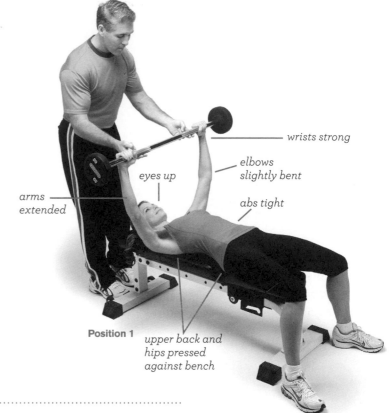

wrists strong

elbows
slightly bent

eyes up

abs tight

arms
extended

Position 1

upper back and
hips pressed
against bench

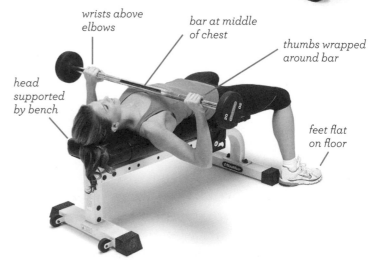

wrists above
elbows

bar at middle
of chest

thumbs wrapped
around bar

head
supported
by bench

feet flat
on floor

Position 2

Too hard? Tone it down
- Decrease the weight on the barbell.
- Bring the barbell down only a quarter of the way.
- Perform this exercise on the floor. This limits how far you can lower the bar, because your elbows will touch the floor.
- Perform this exercise for a shorter amount of time.

Too easy? Kick it up
- Increase the weight on the barbell.
- If you want to get rid of "jiggle arms," move your hands closer together when holding the bar. This places a greater challenge on the backs of your arms (triceps).
- Perform an Incline Bench Press. If you're working out on an adjustable bench, change the angle to increase the difficulty of this movement.
- Perform this exercise for a longer period of time.

TAKE 10 TIPS

Keep your chest up and breathe deeply throughout the exercise. Remember to maintain a solid grip on the bar. It should rest on the bases of your palms at all times. Keep your wrists strong throughout the exercise. Keep your feet on the floor, with your weight on your heels. Your upper back, shoulders and hips should be firmly pressed against the bench at all times.

Barbell Row

EQUIPMENT: **Barbell with weights**

MUSCLES WORKED: **Upper and lower back, shoulders, arms (biceps), core**

This is a wonderful exercise to help strengthen your upper and lower back as well as your shoulders, biceps and abs. It's especially challenging because your body is bent over. Please be sure to read through all the instructions first.

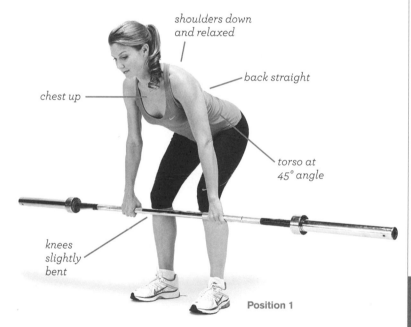

shoulders down and relaxed

back straight

chest up

torso at 45° angle

knees slightly bent

Position 1

❯ GET STARTED

Position your feet shoulder-width apart with your barbell on the floor. Grasp the barbell with your hands wider than shoulder-width apart. Bend your upper body forward from the waist with your torso at a 45° angle. Look at a spot a few feet in front of you, as you relax your shoulders and bend your knees slightly. (**Position 1**)

❯ GET MOVING

1. Begin this exercise by moving the barbell out in front of your knees. Bend your knees, tighten your abdominal muscles, bend your elbows, draw your shoulder blades together, and pull the barbell up toward your belly button. Make sure your knees are positioned inside your arms when you pull up. Your lower back will be slightly arched. Look ahead as you lift (looking down will automatically cause you to round your back). (**Position 2**) Focus on pulling your elbows back, instead of just pulling with your biceps.

LEVEL III

2. Perform this exercise as many times as you can for up to 1 minute.

Too hard? Tone it down

- If you're having a tough time staying in position, perform this exercise with your butt pressed up against a wall. This will help you stay in the same position without standing up straight.
- Decrease the weight on the barbell.
- Go up only a quarter of the way toward your belly button.
- Perform this motion for a shorter amount of time.

Too easy? Kick it up

- Reverse your grip. Hold the bar with your palms facing up.
- Increase the weight on the barbell.
- Perform this motion for a longer period of time.

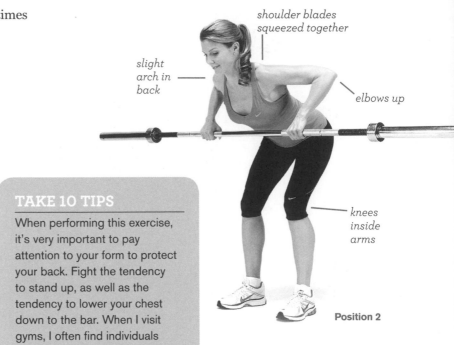

shoulder blades squeezed together

slight arch in back

elbows up

knees inside arms

Position 2

TAKE 10 TIPS

When performing this exercise, it's very important to pay attention to your form to protect your back. Fight the tendency to stand up, as well as the tendency to lower your chest down to the bar. When I visit gyms, I often find individuals doing this exercise incorrectly—looking down, rounding their backs or straightening their legs.

Barbell Shoulder Press and Front Squat

EQUIPMENT: Barbell with weights
MUSCLES WORKED: Shoulders, legs, butt, arms and core

This is a champ of an exercise! You'll be performing a shoulder press and then a front squat with a barbell. Combining these two movements really gets your heart pumping, as well as toning and strengthening your shoulders, legs, butt and core, and helping you with your balance.

❯ GET STARTED

Looking straight ahead, stand with your chest up, feet shoulder-width apart and knees slightly bent, holding the barbell by letting it rest on the bases of your upraised palms. Position the barbell in front of your shoulders, near your clavicle. (**Position 1**)

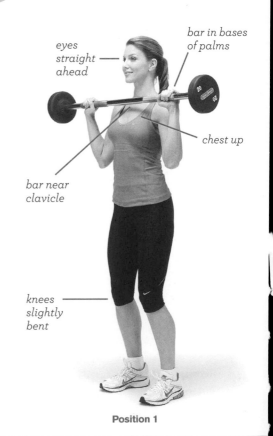

eyes straight ahead

bar in bases of palms

chest up

bar near clavicle

knees slightly bent

Position 1

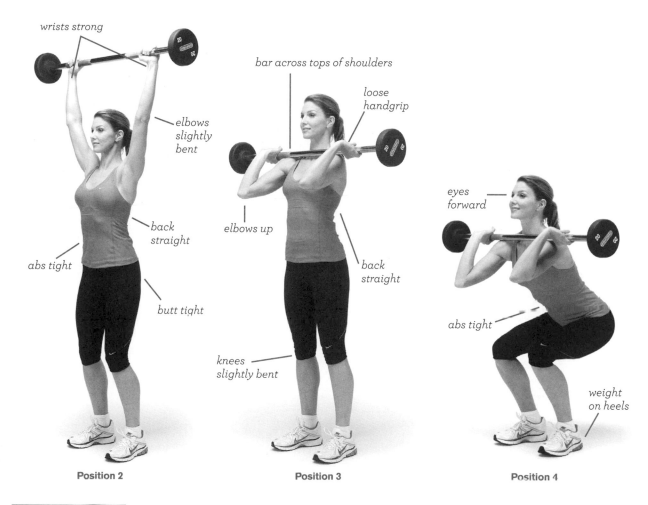

wrists strong

elbows slightly bent

back straight

abs tight

butt tight

Position 2

bar across tops of shoulders

loose handgrip

elbows up

back straight

knees slightly bent

Position 3

eyes forward

abs tight

weight on heels

Position 4

▶ GET MOVING

1. Keeping your abdominal muscles tight and your wrists strong, press the barbell overhead. Extend your arms with a slight bend in your elbows. (**Position 2**) Slowly lower the bar back down to shoulder level. Tighten the muscles of your buttocks—this helps to avoid arching your back. This is the shoulder press part of the exercise.

2. Now position the barbell on top of your shoulders, in front. Hold the bar with a loose grip; your shoulders support the weight of the barbell, not your hands. Before doing the squat, raise your elbows, with your upper arms almost parallel to the floor. Position your feet with your toes pointing out. Your knees should be slightly bent. (**Position 3**)

3. Keeping your abdominals tight and your back strong, sit back into a squat position by slowly lowering your weight down as if you were going to sit in a chair. Keep your elbows up and your eyes looking forward. Be sure you don't extend your knee over your toes when going down in your squat. Go down as low as you comfortably can. This is the squat part of the exercise. (**Position 4**)

4. Next, push your weight up to a standing position, pressing from your heels. Keep your chin parallel to the ground, elbows up, while continuing to hold the bar with your shoulders and hands.

5. Perform as many shoulder presses and front squat repetitions as you can in 1 minute.

Too hard? Tone it down
- Decrease the weight on the barbell.
- Rest between repetitions.
- Perform this exercise for a shorter time frame.

Too easy? Kick it up
- Increase the weight on the barbell.
- Descend lower in the squat.
- Perform the motion for longer than 1 minute.

> **TAKE 10 TIPS**
>
> When performing the shoulder press and the front squat, keep your back strong and abs tight. Remember to look straight ahead—looking down can affect your form and technique for both motions. Also, when performing the front squat, keep your elbows pressed up and your hand grip loose as you rest the bar on your shoulders; this will help you maintain a proper back position. And be sure to breathe comfortably throughout the exercise.

② minutes | Core-Strengthening Exercises

Barbell Twist

EQUIPMENT: Barbell with weights
MUSCLES WORKED: Shoulders, arms and core

I love twisting motions because they mimic what we all do on a daily basis. Whether you're lifting groceries out of the van, turning around to grab something in the back seat or simply moving a box out of the attic, it's important to have strong core muscles to perform the daily tasks of life.

▶ GET STARTED

Start with the barbell in a vertical position with one end on the floor, where it will be stationary (for example, on top of a weight plate or in the corner of the room). Stand 1 to 2 feet away from the barbell with your feet shoulder-width apart. Hold the bar securely with one hand on top of the other (below the weight) and extend your arms. Your back should be straight and your knees slightly bent. (**Position 1**)

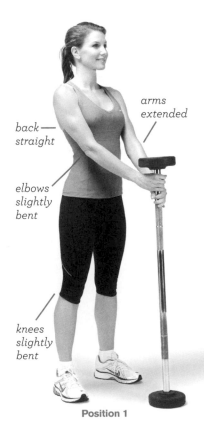

back straight

arms extended

elbows slightly bent

knees slightly bent

Position 1

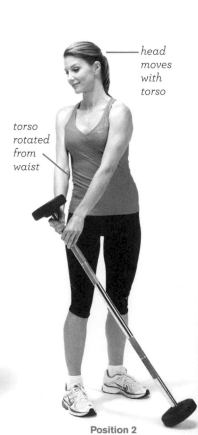

head moves with torso

torso rotated from waist

Position 2

▶ GET MOVING

1. Slowly begin to rotate your torso, using your waist (oblique) muscles to twist to the right with your arms fully extended. (Your hands are still holding the barbell.) Keep your back straight and make sure your head moves with your torso. (**Position 2**)

2. Now rotate to the other side.

3. Perform this exercise as many times as you can, alternating from side to side, for up to 1 minute.

Too hard? Tone it down
- Stand closer to the bar.
- Bend your elbows more throughout the exercise.
- Decrease the weight on the barbell.
- Perform the movement for less than 1 minute.

Too easy? Kick it up
- Position your feet farther away from the bar.
- Use a longer barbell.
- Increase the weight on the barbell.

- Variation: Squat down when performing the exercise.
- Perform the movement for longer than 1 minute.

> **TAKE 10 TIPS**
>
> To get the most out of this movement, use the muscles of your waist (not your arms) to rotate in each direction. Breathe comfortably throughout the exercise.

Barbell Back Extension

EQUIPMENT: Barbell and weights

MUSCLES WORKED: Upper and lower back, butt and backs of legs (hamstrings)

One very important tip here: Think of this exercise as sitting back with your butt and hips (pushing your butt back), with a straight and strong back rather than simply bending over.

▶ GET STARTED

Stand with your back straight, feet hip-width apart and knees slightly bent, holding the barbell below your waist, with your arms extended and palms facing your body, shoulder-width apart. (**Position 1**)

▶ GET MOVING

1. To keep your back straight, press your hips and butt back instead of bending over with your back rounded. Tighten your abdominal muscles and bend over from the waist, lowering the bar to a comfortable level.

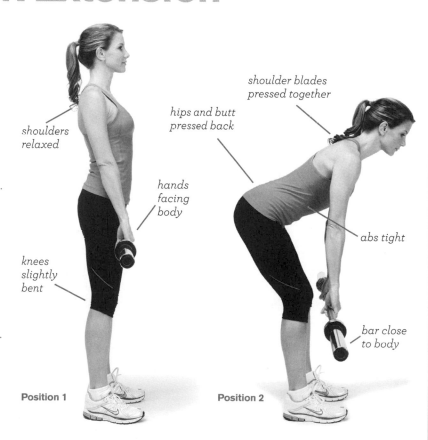

shoulders relaxed

hands facing body

knees slightly bent

Position 1

shoulder blades pressed together

hips and butt pressed back

abs tight

bar close to body

Position 2

LEVEL III

You don't have to go too far with this exercise to make it effective. Keep your shoulders back and down. (**Position 2**)

2. Moving slowly and under control, perform this up-and-down movement as many times as you can for up to 1 minute.

Too hard? Tone it down
- Decrease the weight on the barbell.
- Lower the bar down only a quarter of the way.
- Perform the movement for less than 1 minute.

Too easy? Kick it up
- Increase the weight on the barbell.
- Lower the bar farther down.
- Perform the movement longer than 1 minute.

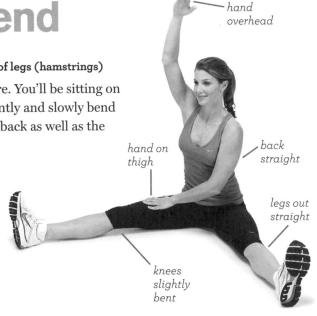

Position 1

TAKE 10 TIPS

Think of this movement as a hamstring stretch as opposed to a lower back exercise. Think of gently and slowly stretching the hamstrings as you lower the weight down, pressing your hips and butt back while keeping the bar close to your body. Also, be sure your head is moving in alignment with your body. Keep your head slightly up when sitting back and lowering the weight down.

---

① minute | Stretching and Deep Breathing

Seated Side Bend

EQUIPMENT: None

MUSCLES WORKED: Upper and lower back and backs of legs (hamstrings)

You can do this relaxing stretch anytime, anywhere. You'll be sitting on the floor with your legs spread apart while you gently and slowly bend over to one side, stretching your upper and lower back as well as the backs of your legs.

▶ GET STARTED

Sitting on the floor, extend your legs straight out to the sides as far as you comfortably can with your knees slightly bent. Sit up straight. Position your left hand on top of your right thigh and reach your right arm overhead (as if you were asking a question in class). (**Position 1**)

hand overhead

hand on thigh

back straight

legs out straight

knees slightly bent

▶ GET MOVING

1. Slowly lean your upper body and right arm to the left, lowering your torso to the side, bending from the waist. As you lean to the side, keep looking straight ahead and allow your head to move in alignment with your upper body. Stretch to mild tension and hold for 15 seconds. (**Position 2**)

2. Reverse your arms and stretch to the other side for another 15 seconds.

Too hard? Tone it down
- Perform this stretch while seated in a chair.
- Don't lean so far over to the side; increase inch by inch over time.
- Hold this stretch for a shorter period of time.

Too easy? Kick it up
- Make your stretch deeper.
- Place your legs farther apart.
- Hold the stretch for a longer period of time.

TAKE 10 TIPS

To get the most out of this stretch, sit up tall with your body elongated, and keep your shoulders relaxed and square as you lean to one side. Also, remember to allow your head to move with your upper body. Move slowly and under control, and breathe deeply throughout the stretch.

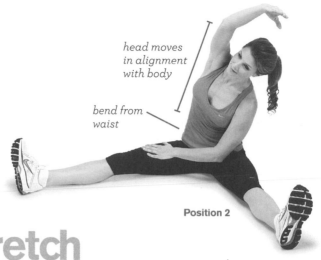

head moves in alignment with body

bend from waist

Position 2

Lengthening Stretch

EQUIPMENT: None

MUSCLES WORKED: Core, back, shoulders, arms and legs

You're going to like the last stretch. It's very simple, but it's also one of the most relaxing stretches you will perform.

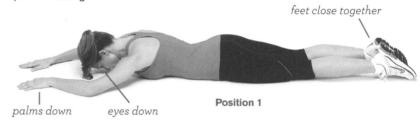

feet close together

palms down   *eyes down*

Position 1

▶ GET STARTED

Lie down on your stomach, looking down, with your feet close together, your face near the floor and your arms out in front of you with the palms of your hands flat on the floor. (**Position 1**)

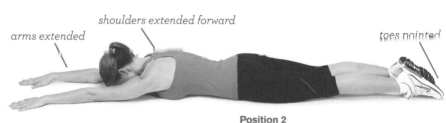

arms extended   *shoulders extended forward*   *toes pointed*

Position 2

▶ GET MOVING

1. Slowly walk your hands away from your shoulders, extending your arms as far as you can. Also, elongate your upper and lower body by pointing your toes and straightening your legs. (**Position 2**)

2. Hold the stretch for 30 seconds

Too hard? Tone it down
- Decrease the distance of your stretch.
- Hold the stretch for a shorter period of time.

Too easy? Kick it up
- Increase the distance of your stretch.
- Hold the stretch for a longer period of time.

TAKE 10 TIPS

To get the most out of this stretch, imagine that someone is gently pulling your feet while someone else is slowly pulling your hands and arms, elongating your spine and body. Remember to breathe deeply.

Well done!
You have just completed your third 4•3•2•1 workout at Level III! Feel free to take a break or, if you'd like, go back and repeat portions of this workout or the entire circuit.

LEVEL III

WORKOUT 4

This last workout in the 10-Minute Total Body Breakthrough really mixes it all up. (Don't forget to warm up first!) Workout 4 includes exercises that not only incorporate *all* the various pieces of equipment from this level—a barbell (with weights if you want), dumbbells and a medicine ball—but also use a stability ball and a resistance band. Talk about dynamic!

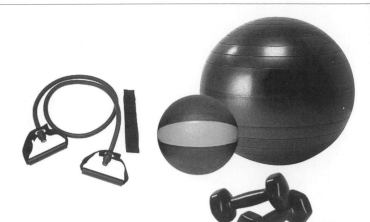

④ minutes | High-Energy Aerobic Training

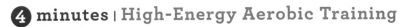

Tuck Jumps and Jogging in Place

EQUIPMENT: None
MUSCLES WORKED: Heart, shoulders, arms, core and legs

Often a tuck jump is done by athletes or cheerleaders jumping high in the sky, tucking their knees up to their chests. Don't let that intimidate you! You don't have to be an athlete or a cheerleader to perform this motion, nor do you have to bring your knees all the way up to your chest. This exercise is simple, but it impacts every muscle group in your body.

❯ GET STARTED

Begin this motion by standing tall with your back straight, your arms at your sides, your shoulders relaxed and your feet positioned hip-width apart. (**Position 1**)

❯ GET MOVING

1. Lean forward slightly and jump explosively up in the air while simultaneously throwing your arms in front of you up to shoulder level. While you're in the air, tuck your knees toward your chest. (**Position 2**) Straighten your legs and land on the balls of your feet so you can jump right back up again. (**Position 3**)

2. Perform Tuck Jumps at a leisurely pace to warm up your body. Keep your back straight and your weight on the balls of your feet. Move under control throughout this movement as you keep up this pace for 30 seconds.

3. Next, begin your Jogging in Place movements at a moderate pace (see page 137). After the 30 seconds of light jogging is up, get ready for another set of Tuck Jumps.

LEVEL III

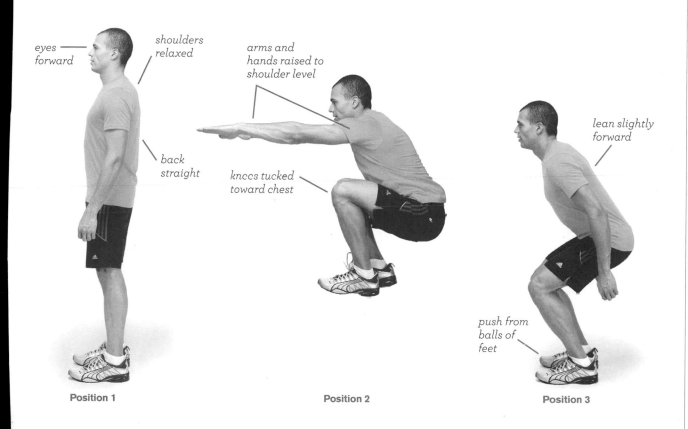

eyes forward

shoulders relaxed

arms and hands raised to shoulder level

back straight

knees tucked toward chest

lean slightly forward

push from balls of feet

Position 1

Position 2

Position 3

4. Keep alternating Jogging in Place with Tuck Jumps every 30 seconds for a total of 4 minutes. See if your jogging can progressively become a little faster and your Tuck Jumps can get quite a bit faster. The first couple of minutes should be used to warm up your body, so remember to ease into your workout, increasing your pace as you progress through the 4 minutes.

Too hard? Tone it down
- Move slower throughout the exercise.
- Don't jump as high when performing the Tuck Jumps.
- Keep your hands on your hips throughout both motions.
- Instead of Jogging in Place, do Marching in Place (see page 103).
- Perform fewer repetitions.
- Perform the exercise for a shorter period of time.

Too easy? Kick it up
- Move faster throughout the exercise.
- Bring your knees closer to your chest during your Tuck Jumps.
- Jump as high and as quickly as you can.
- Throw your arms up higher and with greater force when performing your Tuck Jumps.
- Hold a medicine ball overhead when performing your Tuck Jumps.
- Perform the exercise for a longer period of time.

TAKE 10 TIPS

During your Tuck Jumps, think of being "light on your feet" and avoid landing on your heels. Don't worry about jumping too high. In time, you'll be able to increase the height and speed of your jumps.

LEVEL III

3 minutes | Resistance Exercise

Barbell Overhead Squat

EQUIPMENT: **Barbell with weights**
MUSCLES WORKED: **Legs, butt, arms, shoulders and core**

This is same as the Band Overhead Squat you learned in Workout 4 of Level II (see page 173), but with a twist! Now you'll be holding a barbell over your head throughout the motion. This variation provides a greater challenge to your upper and lower body as well as your core. Try this exercise with just the bar, before adding any weights, to ensure you're doing it correctly.

❯GET STARTED

Hold a barbell with both hands on top of your shoulders with your hands wider than shoulder-width apart and palms facing away from your body. Stand up tall, shoulder blades squeezed together, with your feet shoulder-width apart. Next, press the barbell up over your head, extending both arms with your elbows slightly bent. This is your starting position. (**Position 1**)

❯GET MOVING

1. Keeping the barbell above and slightly behind your head, look straight ahead, keep your chest up, tighten your abdominal muscles and sit back into a squat position, slowly lowering your weight down as if you were going to sit in a chair. As with all other squat motions, be sure your knees don't extend over your toes when in the squat position. Also, keep your head in alignment with your torso. Go down as low as you comfortably can. (**Position 2**) It's natural to lean forward slightly from the waist to maintain your balance, due to the weight of the barbell; resist that temptation and push your arms and shoulders back as you lower down into the squat position.

2. Next, tighten the muscles of your buttocks and push up to a standing position by pressing from your heels—all the while keeping your arms extended and the barbell over your head, with your elbows slightly bent. Keep your shoulders relaxed, your chest up and your wrists firm and strong.

3. Perform this exercise, with the barbell overhead, as many times as you can for up to 1 minute.

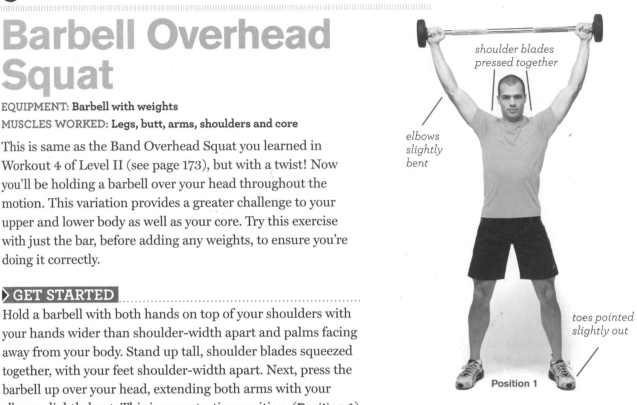

shoulder blades pressed together

elbows slightly bent

toes pointed slightly out

Position 1

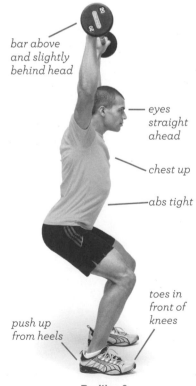

bar above and slightly behind head

eyes straight ahead

chest up

abs tight

toes in front of knees

push up from heels

Position 2